Autologous
Stem Cell Transplants

A Handbook for Patients

Autologous Stem Cell Transplants

A Handbook for Patients

By Susan K. Stewart

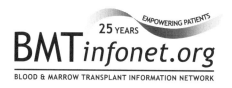

BLOOD & MARROW TRANSPLANT INFORMATION NETWORK

1548 Old Skokie Rd, Unit 1, Highland Park, IL 60035
phone: 847-433-3313   toll-free: 888-597-7674
email: help@bmtinfonet.org
bmtinfonet.org

Copyright 2000, Revised 2012, 2014, 2019

ISBN 978-1-7337268-0-1

Publication of this book was made possible, in part, by a generous gift from

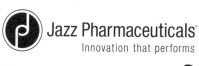

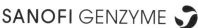

Other books written by Susan K. Stewart:

Bone Marrow and Blood Stem Cell Transplants:
A Guide for Patients and Their Loved Ones
(for patients undergoing a transplant using donor cells)

Graft-versus-Host Disease
What to Know, What to Do

In Spanish:
Trasplantes de Médula Ósea y de Células Madre Sanguíneas:
Una Guía para Pacientes y sus Seres Queridos

Enfermedad Injerto contra Huésped
Qué necesita saber. Qué necesita hacer.

This book is intended to help you understand bone
marrow, stem cell and cord blood transplantation but
is not a substitute for medical advice from your
healthcare team.

Acknowledgements

Writing this book was not a solo effort. The generosity of many people — doctors, nurses, social workers, transplant survivors, caregivers, my family and friends — is reflected in this book. They patiently shared their time, expertise and personal experiences. Without their help, this book would not have been possible.

Special thanks to:

Patrick J. Stiff MD, who contributed countless hours to the first edition of this book, and who reviewed this new, revised edition.

Martin S. Tallman MD, a warm, caring doctor and a personal friend who supported me first through my transplant, and afterwards as a medical advisor on this book.

Jan Sugar, who helped write and edit several sections of this book.

Norm Bendell, whose illustrations appear throughout the book. Thanks, Norm, for helping us to lighten up a very difficult text.

Our scientific advisors for this edition:

Stephanie Lee MD, MPH, Fred Hutchinson Cancer Research Center

Navneet Majhail MD, MS, Cleveland Clinic

Jayesh Mehta MD, Northwestern Memorial Hospital and Northwestern University

Kenneth Miller MD, Tufts Medical Center

Marcie Riches MD, MS, The University of North Carolina

Scott Rowley MD, Medstar Georgetown University Hospital and Hackensack University Medical Center

Patrick Stiff MD, Loyola University Medical Center

Keith Sullivan MD, Duke University Medical Center

Kim Kultgen, our graphic artist, who worked tirelessly on this book to make it a pleasure to read.

The transplant survivors and caregivers quoted throughout the book who gave it life. They have journeyed down the transplant path and have generously shared their experience and insights.

BMT InfoNet staff members Marla O'Keefe, Lynne Spina, Cindy Kessler and Michala O'Brien who helped edit drafts of this book.

And finally, to my husband and son whose patience and support helped make this book possible.

This book is dedicated
to
Ruth Krueger
My mother, mentor and constant source of support

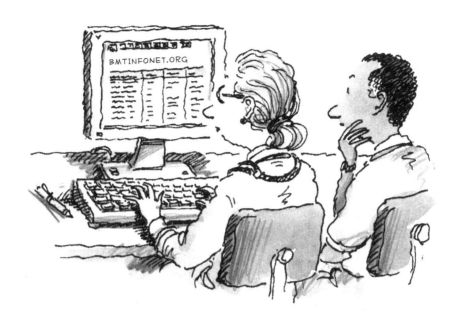

Visit bmtinfonet.org

Our website is your gateway to detailed information about what to expect before, during and after your transplant. Popular features include:

- **Transplant Basics:** how to prepare for transplant and manage challenges that arise during and after transplant

- **Emotional support** for patients, survivors and caregivers

- **Facts about nearly 200 transplant centers** including staff, number of transplants performed, accreditation and diseases treated

- **Video Learning Library** presentations about the medical, psychosocial and financial challenges associated with transplant

- **Resource Directory** with links to financial help, disease information and more

You can also phone us toll-free at 888-597-7674.

We're with you every step of the way!

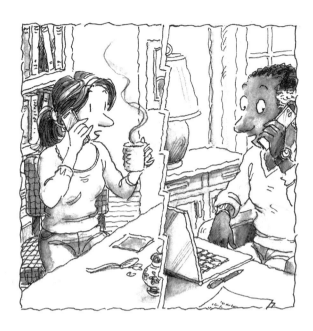

BMT InfoNet
Caring Connections Program

If you or a loved one is going to have a transplant, chances are you are feeling scared and overwhelmed.

BMT InfoNet's **Caring Connections Program** can help.

Talk with people who:
- have been through a transplant
- understand how you feel
- can provide non-medical information and emotional support
- can offer tips for coping with household and job responsibilities, the needs of other family members and more

If you are a family member of a patient, you can use the Caring Connections program too!

Request a Caring Connection by phoning 888-597-7674 or online at bmtinfonet.org/caring-connection.

Table of Contents

Dear Friend,

In 1988, after being diagnosed with leukemia, my doctor recommended an autologous bone marrow transplant. I'd never before heard of a bone marrow or stem cell transplant.

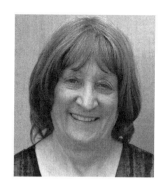

I was confused and overwhelmed. All the medical terms used to describe the treatment were new to me. Often, I couldn't even figure out the right questions to ask!

After recovering from my transplant, I met other survivors and learned my experience was not unique. So, I wrote this book to help you understand the complex medical information you'll receive before, during and after your transplant.

There's no getting around it. Autologous transplantation is a confusing subject. There's a lot of information to absorb in this book. Take it at your own pace.

If you only want the basics, start with Chapters One and Two. Then use the Table of Contents and Index to find answers to the questions that concern you most. When you are ready for more details, read the other chapters that thoroughly discuss each step of the transplant process.

Throughout the book you will find quotations from transplant survivors and family caregivers — real people who faced the same challenges that now lie before you. They will tell you firsthand what it feels like to undergo and survive an autologous stem cell transplant.

I know how difficult it is to make the decision to have a transplant, undergo the treatment and get back to a normal life. I hope this book helps make your experience a little easier.

Sue Stewart

Susan Stewart
Executive Director, BMT InfoNet

Chapter One

HISTORY OF TRANSPLANTATION

When I was first diagnosed with leukemia, I got very little encouragement from my local oncologist. Back then, bone marrow transplants weren't so common. He really tried to discourage me. He said 'A transplant is not for you. You might as well give up.' It felt pretty good to come home after my transplant, a survivor.

Jean Durko, 17-year transplant survivor

Bone marrow, peripheral blood stem cell and umbilical cord blood transplantation are medical procedures used to treat people with diseases once thought incurable. Patients with diseases such as multiple myeloma, lymphoma, Hodgkin lymphoma, autoimmune and genetic diseases and some solid tumors may be a candidate for an autologous transplant.

The technical name for bone marrow, peripheral blood stem cell and cord blood transplantation is hematopoietic cell transplantation.

Types of Transplants

There are three types of transplant: allogeneic (al-o-je-náy-ik), syngeneic (sin-je-náy-ik) and autologous (aw-tól-o-gus).

Allogeneic transplantation — a transplant that uses cells from a donor — is typically used to treat people who have a bone marrow disorder such as leukemia or aplastic anemia. In this procedure, the diseased bone marrow is destroyed by high-dose chemotherapy and/

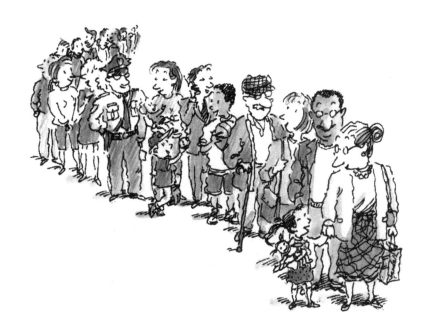

or radiation and replaced with blood stem cells provided by a donor.

Syngeneic transplantation is similar to allogeneic transplantation in that the stem cells come from another person. The difference is that the donor is an identical twin, rather than another relative or an unrelated donor.

Autologous transplantation — the type of transplant discussed in this book — is much more common today than allogeneic transplantation and involves fewer potential complications. In this procedure, the person's own stem cells are collected and stored. The patient then undergoes high-dose chemotherapy and/or radiation to destroy the disease. Since the high-dose chemotherapy and radiation also destroy healthy blood cells, the previously collected stem cells are re-infused into the patient to rescue him or her from this life-threatening side-effect.

A Historical Perspective

The first serious attempts to transplant bone marrow into humans occurred in the late 1950s. Although several patients achieved a remission after transplant (there was no evidence of disease), most of them relapsed (the disease came back) shortly thereafter.

In the early 1960's, two successful transplants occurred using bone marrow donated by an identical twin: one in the U.S. and the other in China. Both patients were children with a blood disorder called severe aplastic anemia and were cured following their transplant

The first successful bone marrow transplant using marrow donated by a sibling who was **not** an identical twin took place in 1968. The patient was a baby boy who was born with an immune deficiency disease that had taken the life of all eleven male children born on his mother's side of the family. After two transplants, the child returned home and grew to be a healthy adult.

Similar successes soon were reported for patients with leukemia. By 1986, hundreds of transplant centers worldwide were performing 5,000 transplants annually.

Unfortunately, many patients who could have benefited from a bone marrow transplant could not undergo the procedure because they did not have a sibling with a matching tissue type. In 1973, two teams of doctors overcame this obstacle:

- one in London, who successfully transplanted marrow from an unrelated donor into a child who had chronic granulomatous disease (CGD)

- and the second, in New York, where doctors did seven transplants with marrow from an unrelated donor for a child with severe combined immunodeficiency disease (SCIDS).

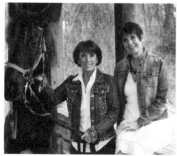

Nancy King McLain and her twin sister and donor, Bonnie Engesmoe

Nancy King McLain, the longest living transplant survivor, underwent a bone marrow transplant with marrow from her twin sister Bonnie in 1963. Currently, Nancy is a retired teacher who enjoys riding, skating, cycling, swimming and skiing.

"I love life every day because I know how close I was to losing it at such an early age," says Nancy.

In 1986, the National Marrow Donor Registry® (now called the Be The Match Registry®) was established to facilitate more transplants with unrelated donors.

It was not until the late 1980s that autologous transplants became widely used. In 1978, researchers reported several successful autologous transplants in patients with lymphoma. By 1990, more autologous transplants were being performed than allogeneic transplants. An estimated 30,000 autologous transplants are now performed each year worldwide — more than 14,000 per year in the United States.

Diseases Treated by Transplant

More than two dozen different diseases can now be treated with an autologous transplant. Those treated most often are multiple myeloma, lymphoma, Hodgkin lymphoma and neuroblastoma.

The likelihood that an autologous transplant will succeed hinges on several factors. The patient must be healthy enough to withstand the rigors of a transplant. The disease must be sensitive to the particular combination of high-dose chemotherapy and/or radiation given prior to transplant. The transplant team must be skilled at spotting and managing complications that can arise from the treatment.

Although not all patients are cured by an autologous transplant, it can prolong and improve a patient's quality of life for many years.

A Look into the Future

There is considerable, promising research underway to improve upon the results now being achieved with autologous transplantation. Some investigators are testing new combinations of high-dose chemotherapy to determine which is most effective in destroying a particular disease. Others are investigating ways to make the patient's own immune system get rid of diseased cells that may remain after transplantation. Still others are exploring ways to prevent complications associated with the treatment.

Many people with diseases once thought incurable are now leading productive lives, thanks to progress made in the field of autologous stem cell transplantation.

Chapter Two

AN INTRODUCTION TO TRANSPLANTATION

I still find it bizarre that I would be the one to get so sick. I was very physically active. I rode my bike 2,000 miles a year, swam about 100 miles and was active in my children's lives. Cancer happens to people you read about in the newspaper. It doesn't strike an enormously healthy, happy and vital 39-year-old family man.

Mike Eckhardt, 11-year transplant survivor

This chapter will give you a broad overview of autologous transplantation. More detailed information about autologous transplantation can be found in the remaining chapters of this book.

What are Bone Marrow and Blood Stem Cells?

Bone marrow is a spongy tissue found inside bones. Bone marrow contains blood stem cells — special cells that generate most of the body's blood cells. Blood stem cells produce:

- white blood cells (leukocytes) to fight infection

- red blood cells (erythrocytes) to carry oxygen to and remove carbon dioxide from organs and tissues

- and platelets which enable blood to clot

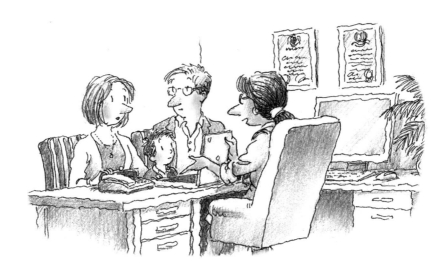

If you are considering an autologous transplant, you may want to familiarize yourself with the different types of blood cells and their functions. During your treatment, the medical team will count and refer to these different blood cells frequently. (For a detailed discussion of blood cells, go to Appendix A, About Blood Cells.)

Why an Autologous Transplant?

Sometimes a patient cannot be cured with standard dosages of chemotherapy or radiation. High-dose chemotherapy and/or radiation may cure the patient, but will also destroy the stem cells that create blood cells. Without these blood cells, the body cannot fight infection, get oxygen to tissues or allow blood to clot.

An autologous transplant lets doctors rescue a patient from the life-threatening side effects of high-dose chemotherapy/radiation therapy. Stem cells are collected from the patient's bone marrow or bloodstream before the high-dose chemotherapy and/or radiation, and are reinfused after treatment. An autologous stem cell transplant is sometimes called an autologous stem cell rescue.

Sources of Stem Cells

The earliest autologous transplants were bone marrow transplants. Bone marrow is rich in the stem cells that produce the various types of blood cells.

In the mid-1980s, researchers discovered that stem cells could be moved out of the bone marrow into the bloodstream where they could be collected and used successfully in an autologous transplant. Stem cells collected from the bloodstream are called peripheral blood stem cells.

Who Can Undergo Autologous Transplantation?

To be a candidate for an autologous transplant, you must be healthy enough to tolerate the transplant procedure. Age, general physical condition, diagnosis, the stage of the disease and prior treatment are all considered by your physician to determine whether you are a good candidate for an autologous transplant.

Tests of your heart, lungs, kidneys and other vital organs will be performed prior to transplant to ensure you can tolerate the procedure. If a tumor is present, its status will be evaluated at this time. The tests for organ function and tumor status are later used as a baseline against which post-transplant tests can be compared.

Stem Cell Collection/Harvest

Prior to the high-dose chemotherapy and/or radiation, your blood stem cells will be collected. If the stem cells are collected from the bloodstream, the procedure is called a peripheral blood stem cell

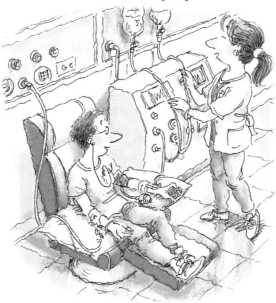

collection or harvest. The collection is usually done in the outpatient clinic and is not a surgical procedure.

The blood stem cells may be collected from a vein in your arm, or through a device called a central venous catheter that is inserted into a large vein in your chest under local anesthesia. The catheter makes it possible to collect stem cells without inserting needles into your hands or arms. Later, the catheter may be used to give you chemotherapy, other drugs and fluids, and to withdraw blood samples painlessly. You may also hear the catheter referred to as a central line, Groshong®, Hickman® or apheresis catheter.

Prior to the stem cell harvest, you will receive daily injections of a drug such as filgrastim (Neupogen®) and/or plerixafor (Mozobil®) which moves stem cells out of the bone marrow into the bloodstream where they can be collected. Some patients also receive a small dosage of chemotherapy before the harvest to help move stem cells into the bloodstream and to shrink their tumor.

The medicines used to move the stem cells from your bone marrow into your bloodstream can cause aching and some discomfort in your lower back and hips. This pain is similar to the body aches you may experience with a viral infection like the flu.

During the harvest, which can last two-to-six hours, you will sit in a comfortable chair. Blood will be withdrawn from a vein in your arm or through the catheter in your chest, and passed through flexible tubing to an apheresis machine. The machine will remove the stem cells and return the rest of your blood to you. The stem cells are then cryopreserved (frozen at very low temperatures) until the day of transplant.

It usually takes one-to-three days to collect enough stem cells for transplant. In some cases, additional stem cells may be collected and frozen for use at a future date.

You may feel light headed, cold or numb around the lips during the collection. Some patients experience cramping in their hands that is caused by a blood-thinning agent used during the collection procedure. The cramping usually resolves after treatment with calcium supplements. Other possible short-term side effects include bone pain, headache, fatigue and nausea.

Under proper conditions, stem cells can be stored for years and still be viable for transplantation. Your transplant team may ask that you sign a contract detailing how these cells, which are your property, will be stored and under what conditions they can be destroyed.

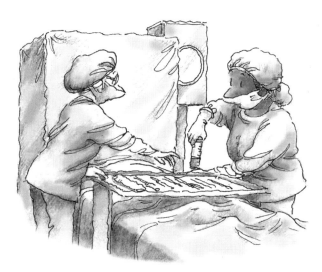

Bone Marrow Harvest

Some patients undergo a bone marrow harvest instead of a stem cell harvest. Occasionally, a patient needs to undergo both in order to collect sufficient stem cells for transplantation.

A bone marrow harvest is a surgical procedure that takes place in a hospital operating room. While you are under general anesthesia, needles are inserted into your rear hip bone where a large quantity of bone marrow is located. The bone marrow, a thick red liquid, is extracted with the needles and syringes. The bone marrow is then frozen until the day of transplant.

Several skin punctures on each hip and multiple bone punctures are required to extract sufficient bone marrow for transplantation. There are no surgical incisions or stitches involved.

The amount of bone marrow harvested depends on your weight and the concentration of stem cells in your marrow. Usually, one-to-two quarts of marrow and blood are harvested. While this may sound like a lot, your body will replace it within four weeks.

When the anesthesia wears off, you may feel some discomfort at the harvest site. The pain will be similar to that associated with a hard fall on the ice and can usually be controlled with acetaminophen (Tylenol®). Patients typically resume normal activities in a few days, although climbing stairs or sitting in one place for a long period of time may be uncomfortable for a week or so.

Conditioning/Preparative Regimen

After the stem cell or bone marrow harvest, you will undergo several days of chemotherapy and/or radiation to destroy your disease. This is called the conditioning or preparative regimen. The exact dosage and combination of chemotherapy and/or radiation varies according to your disease and the protocol (preferred treatment plan) of the transplant team. The conditioning regimen usually lasts four-to-ten days. (For more on this topic, see Chapter Seven, Conditioning/ Preparative.)

Most chemotherapy drugs are given through a thin flexible tube called a central venous catheter (also called a Groshong® or Hickman® catheter, or a central line). The catheter is surgically implanted into a large vein in the chest, just above the heart. It enables the medical staff to give you drugs and blood products painlessly, and to withdraw the many blood samples required during the course of treatment without inserting needles in your arms. The catheter may be left in place for several months after transplant until recovery is complete. Some transplant centers use a catheter inserted into your arm, called a PICC line, for this purpose instead.

Day of Transplant

One-to-three days after the conditioning regimen, the transplant occurs. The stem cells collected from the bloodstream or bone marrow will be infused into you through your catheter. This procedure typically takes 30 minutes to an hour, and is usually done in your hospital room.

You will be awake and may be lightly sedated during the transplant. You will be checked frequently for signs of fever, chills, hives and chest pains. When the transplant is done, the days and weeks of waiting begin.

Engraftment

The two-to-three week period after transplant is a critical time. The conditioning regimen will have destroyed your stem cells, temporarily crippling your immune system. Until the transplanted stem cells begin producing new healthy blood cells, you will be very susceptible to infection and excessive bleeding.

You may be given drugs called growth factors to speed recovery of your blood counts. You'll receive multiple blood transfusions and antibiotics, as needed, to help prevent and fight infection. Platelet transfusions may be needed to help prevent bleeding.

Precautions will be taken to minimize your exposure to viruses and bacteria. Medical personnel will wash their hands with antiseptic soap or alcohol gels. You may be required to wear a mask when you leave the clinic or the hospital room. The mask provides a barrier against bacteria and viruses and reminds others that you are at high risk of developing an infection.

During this period, you may be instructed to avoid fresh vegetables, fruits, plants and cut flowers, since these items can carry bacteria that can cause a serious infection. You may also be told to avoid young children and certain pets until your immune system is functioning normally. (For more on infections see Chapter Eight, Infection.)

Daily blood samples will be taken during this period to determine whether the stem cells have begun producing healthy blood cells. When blood counts begin to rise, the antibiotics and blood and platelet transfusions are generally no longer needed. Once the stem cells are producing a sufficient number of healthy blood cells, you will be discharged from the hospital or outpatient center, provided no other complications have developed.

Where Treatment is Given

Historically, patients were hospitalized during the conditioning regimen, the transplant and the first few weeks of the recovery period. Now, many centers attempt to perform all or part of the treatment in an outpatient facility.

Patients typically spend four-to-twelve hours a day at the outpatient facility during the conditioning regimen and transplant. Following the transplant, you will visit the outpatient facility daily to receive blood and platelet transfusions, intravenous fluids, antinausea medications and antibiotics. At night, you will return home, or to an apartment or hotel room near the hospital, where you will be watched carefully by a family member or a friend who has been trained as your caregiver. (For more on caregivers, see Chapter Eleven, Family Caregiver.)

Some patients are hospitalized for all or part of their treatment. Hospitalization may be required if you do not have a caregiver to monitor you at home, or have medical problems that need around-the-clock monitoring by the medical staff.

How Patients Feel During Transplant

An autologous transplant is a physically and emotionally taxing procedure for both the patient and family.

After the conditioning regimen, you may feel extremely tired, sick and weak. You may experience nausea, vomiting, fever and diarrhea. Activities like walking, sitting up in bed for long periods of time, reading books, talking on the phone, visiting with friends or even watching TV may require more energy than you have.

Complications such as infection or bleeding can develop after transplant, creating additional discomfort. Mouth sores may make eating and swallowing uncomfortable.

Temporary mental confusion, usually related to the medications, sometimes occurs. This can be quite frightening for you and your family members who may not realize that it's temporary. The medical staff can help you deal with these problems.

Handling Emotional Stress

In addition to the physical discomfort, there's also emotional discomfort. It's common for patients and caregivers to seek out professional help for a period of time to help them cope with the transplant experience.

Some patients find the emotional stress more problematic than the physical discomfort. They must not only handle the fact that they have a life-threatening disease, but many fear the transplant

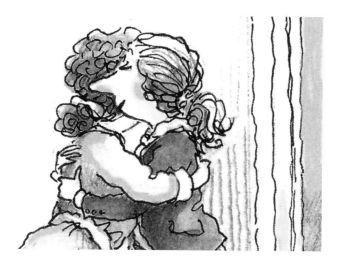

procedure itself. While a transplant offers the hope of a cure or longer life, there are no guarantees. Living with that uncertainty can be very difficult.

Transplant patients can also feel quite isolated. Special precautions taken to guard against infection during recovery sometimes interfere with your ability to interact normally with family and friends. Some friends and family members may not understand, or be poorly equipped to manage the gravity of the situation and the emotional trauma involved in a transplant.

Helplessness is a common feeling among transplant patients and can cause anger or resentment. For many, it is unnerving to be totally dependent on strangers for survival, no matter how competent they may be. Some also find it embarrassing to be dependent on others for help with basic daily functions such as using the bathroom. Trying to decipher unfamiliar medical terms can make the feeling of helplessness worse.

The time spent waiting for blood counts to return to safe levels increases the emotional load. Recovery can be like a roller coaster ride: one day you may feel much better only to awake the next day feeling as sick as ever, even after you have been discharged home. (For more on the emotional aspects of transplant see Chapter Five, Emotional Challenges.)

First Year after Transplant

The length and nature of the recovery period varies from patient to patient. It may take six months or more before you are well enough to resume a normal routine and return to work or school. It is best not to set unrealistic recovery goals or compare your progress to another's. The length of the recovery period is not a good indication of whether or not you have been cured, or how long life has been extended. Some patients simply take longer to recover than others, and can look forward to a long, healthy life.

Sometimes transplant survivors develop an infection or other complication several weeks or months after transplant. If this happens, you may need to be hospitalized for treatment. This can be depressing, since you may be very anxious to put hospital routines behind you. It helps to keep in mind that these setbacks are common and are usually temporary and reversible.

Life during the first year after transplant can be both exhilarating and worrisome. On the one hand, it is exciting to be alive. Many survivors find their quality of life improves after transplant.

Nonetheless, many worry that the disease will come back. It can be many months before one full day passes during which you don't think about your disease or the transplant experience.

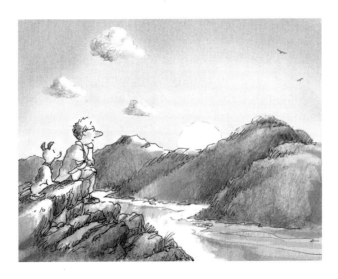

Is It Worth It?

Many survivors say that their quality of life after transplant is as good as or better than before. While autologous stem cell or bone marrow transplants are not always successful, they have cured or prolonged the lives of thousands of people. These survivors are grateful to have been given a new lease on life.

> "Currently, I'm 14 months post-transplant. I celebrated my one-year anniversary by climbing a mountain in Colorado and getting second row seats for a Jimmy Buffet concert. Lots of people celebrated with me and gave me inspirational messages, gifts and support. My favorite gift was from my doctor — an interpretation of my bone marrow biopsy. The interpretation pretty much describes my life today. Normal."

To learn more, visit our website at:

bmtinfonet.org/transplant-basics

Chapter Three

CHOOSING A TRANSPLANT CENTER

Was I scared? I was scared as a rabbit in winter. But I kept thinking, 'there's light at the end of the tunnel and I'm not ready to give up'. I remember the day they put me in the hospital. My 13-year-old son said 'I'm wrapping an invisible rope around you, Mom. Slowly but surely I'm going to tug on it until I get you back home again'. That was the most wonderful thing in the world. I'll never forget that he said that.

Maralyn Collins, 19-year transplant survivor

In the early days of transplantation, autologous transplants were offered by only a handful of medical centers. Today nearly 200 centers perform autologous transplants in the U.S. alone. How do you decide which medical center is best for you?

Depending on your insurance coverage, the choice may be wide open or very limited. In the U.S., many insurers negotiate contracts with a handful of transplant centers and require their plan enrollees to be treated at these centers. Although this limits your choices, the designated medical centers are usually major institutions with a highly experienced transplant team that provides excellent care.

Your particular disease may also limit the number of centers available for consideration. For example, while many centers perform autologous transplants for lymphoma and multiple myeloma, fewer offer transplants for diseases such as amyloidosis.

Your local doctor may recommend a transplant center based on a number of obvious factors, like the transplant team's experience and reputation. Other less obvious factors may include the relationship your doctor has with physicians at the center, and your doctor's prior experience in getting help and information from the center when patients are returned to him or her for follow-up care. Ask why your doctor recommends one center over another, and don't hesitate to ask for an opinion about other transplant centers as well.

BMT InfoNet maintains a list of centers that perform autologous transplants in the United States that includes information on the number of transplants performed, diseases treated, accreditation and contact information. You can access the list at bmtinfonet.org/transplantcenters or by phoning 888-597-7674.

Be The Match® and the Health Resources & Services Administration also have information on transplant centers you may find helpful. Links to these resources are on BMT InfoNet's web site at bmtinfonet.org/choosing-transplant-center.

If you are free to choose between different centers, there are several factors you'll want to consider. The rest of this chapter will explore some of these issues and provide guidance on how to find the center that's right for you.

Accreditation

The Foundation for Accreditation of Cellular Therapy (FACT) inspects transplant programs and accredits those that meet FACT standards. FACT accreditation is a sign that the program has passed a rigorous inspection and is considered by experts in the field to be a quality transplant program.

Go to factwebsite.org to learn which programs are FACT accredited. This information is also included in BMT InfoNet's online transplant center directory at bmtinfonet.org/transplantcenters.

The Transplant Team

When considering a transplant center, focus first on the transplant team — the doctors, nurses, radiologists, pharmacists and other support staff who will be involved in your care. The more training and experience they have in dealing with transplant patients, the better able they'll be to respond to problems. Ask not only about the training and experience of individual team members, but how long they have been working together as a team.

Doctors

FACT standards require that the transplant program director be a licensed physician with board certification in hematology, medical oncology, immunology and/or pediatric hematology/oncology. Some physicians who completed their medical training before 1985 may not be board certified in one of these specialties, but may nonetheless have many years of experience in the field of autologous transplantation. They should be able to provide you with a list of publications they've authored that demonstrate their experience.

The other transplant physicians who will be involved in your care should also be licensed and board certified in one of the specialties described above. Ask if they've had extensive training or experience in the care of transplant patients. Will a transplant physician be on call 24-hours-a-day to handle emergencies and answer questions? If you have a pre-existing medical condition that may complicate your treatment, such as heart or lung problems, ask specifically about the

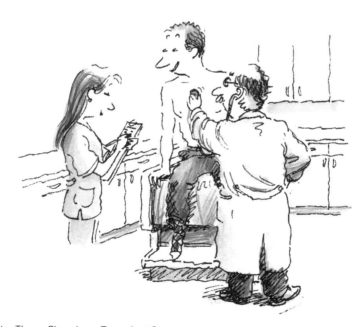

doctors' experience in handling patients with similar problems.

Be sure the transplant team has around-the-clock access to other licensed specialists who may need to be involved in your care. This includes doctors who are board certified in surgery, pulmonary medicine, intensive care, gastroenterology, nephrology, infectious diseases, cardiology, pathology, psychiatry and radiation therapy.

Nurses

A highly trained experienced team of nurses is a critical component of a good transplant program. It's the nurses who will spend the most time with you. They must be able to quickly identify problems and respond appropriately.

Find out how many registered nurses will be involved in your care. Have they been trained and certified in hematology/oncology? How much experience have they had caring for autologous transplant patients? How many nurses per patient are there on the transplant unit?

Psychosocial Support Services

Undergoing an autologous transplant is not only physically difficult, but emotionally taxing as well. Some patients find the emotional trauma more difficult to handle than the physical discomfort. People who have never before sought counseling may need the help

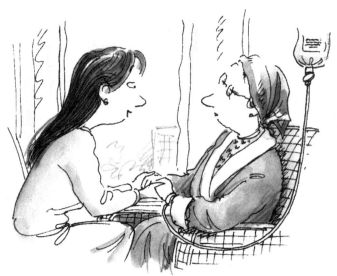

of a psychiatrist, psychologist, social worker or religious counselor to help them cope with the transplant experience.

Psychosocial support services offered by transplant centers vary considerably. Ask whether psychological services will routinely be provided to you or are available upon request. Find out what other programs the transplant center offers to help you and your family cope emotionally such as support groups, yoga, mindfulness and other relaxation techniques.

Pediatric Patients

If the transplant patient is your child, find out whether the doctors, nurses and support staff have training and experience in treating pediatric patients. Children are not just small adults. Their growing bodies may react differently to drugs, and their emotional needs are different as well.

Some transplant centers specialize in treating only pediatric patients, while others treat both children and adults — sometimes with the same staff. If the center you're considering does not limit its practice to pediatric patients, be sure that the team members, as well as consulting specialists, are experienced in caring for pediatric patients.

Some centers have strict guidelines about how long parents can remain with their hospitalized child and require them to leave in the evening. Others will allow parents to remain overnight if they wish. Make sure you're comfortable with the center's guidelines on this matter.

Ask what sort of age-appropriate activities and counseling will be provided to your child during his or her treatment. Inquire about the center's philosophy on providing pain medications before painful procedures such as bone marrow biopsies. Can your child bring favorite toys, clothes, etc. to the hospital room? Rules vary considerably at different centers on these matters, and you should be sure you're comfortable with their approach before your child is admitted. (For more on pediatric transplants see Chapter Six, When Your Child Needs a Transplant.)

Support for Family Caregivers

Many transplant programs now provide some or all of the treatment in the outpatient clinic. This means that a primary family caregiver must be available to carefully monitor and care for the patient when he or she returns home.

Ask what sort of support systems are in place to help family caregivers. Find out what kind of training your caregiver will receive, and whether he or she will have access to volunteers who can help with daily tasks, like shopping or laundry, particularly if the transplant is taking place out of town.

Number of Transplants Performed

Ask how long the transplant center has been performing transplants and how many transplants are performed each year. Although the training and experience of the transplant team members are the most important factors to evaluate, the number of transplants performed by a center can often give you a rough idea of the team's experience. You can find out how many transplants have been performed at a center by inquiring at the center directly, by contacting BMT InfoNet at 888-597-7674 or online at bmtinfonet.org/transplantcenters.

Treatment Plans

The treatment plan or "protocol" for your disease can vary from center to center. The type and dosage of chemotherapy drugs may differ. Some centers may be testing new methods of handling transplant complications. Others may be investigating novel ways to prevent relapse.

The risks associated with various treatment plans may differ as well. Ask what is known about the effectiveness and risks associated with the protocol suggested for you. Find out what will be done to manage the complications, and satisfy yourself that the center has the experience necessary to spot and quickly treat problems when they arise.

You might want to ask how many patients have already undergone the same treatment at that transplant center, how many have developed problems and how many have benefitted from the treatment. Ask the doctor to be as specific as possible in describing how patients that are similar to you (e.g., same age, stage of disease and medical problems) have fared. Keep in mind, however, that such data may not be available for newer treatment plans.

Success Rates

The question asked most often by patients is "Which transplant center has the best success rate?"

A successful transplant can be defined in different ways. It may mean that the stem cells engrafted and the patient did not die of complications while in the hospital. Alternatively, it may mean that the patient lived one, three, five years or more without a recurrence of the disease. When discussing success rates with transplant teams, be sure you understand how they are defining the term.

Many factors influence a center's success rate. A hospital that accepts only prime candidates for transplant — young persons, those in an early stage of their disease and those who have responded well to prior treatment — may report better success rates than centers who treat older or sicker patients.

When asking about success rates, be sure the figure you're given pertains to treatment at that center, using the same protocol and for the same disease. Success rates for patients who were treated with a different protocol may not be a good gauge of how well you'll fare with the treatment plan proposed for you. Success rates from other centers may be better or worse than success rates achievable at the center you're considering.

Financial Considerations

Autologous transplants are very costly, even if insurance is paying for all or most of the procedure. In addition to medical expenses, your family may incur significant travel, lodging and meal expenses, particularly if you are being treated out of town. If your caregiver must take time off from work to be with you, this can add to the financial burden. Additional child care expenditures may be necessary while a parent is being treated.

Talk to the social worker at the transplant center to find out what sort of assistance is available to help with these expenses. Some centers have special arrangements with local hotels or dormitories to house patients and family members at low or no cost. Others can help you apply for financial assistance.

If convincing your insurance company to pay for the transplant is a problem, find out what sort of help the center will provide. Ask how successful the center has been in appealing an insurer's denial of coverage should that occur. (For more on insurance problems see Chapter Four, Insurance and Fundraising.)

If insurance refuses to pay for your treatment, ask what sort of alternative financing arrangements the center is willing to make with you. Most centers will refuse to provide treatment unless insurance pre-approves payment, or the family makes a hefty down payment.

Charges for autologous transplants vary considerably from center to center. A center may not be able to quote an exact price for your treatment, since the cost of your care will depend on whether you need to be hospitalized and any special treatment needs. Do, however, ask for a ballpark estimate of the cost, particularly if you will have to pay for the treatment yourself.

Long-Term Follow-Up

After you leave the transplant center, your care will eventually be turned over to your local doctor, ideally a specialist like an oncologist or hematologist. Since most doctors have not received specific training in the care of transplant patients, it's important that the transplant center staff be accessible to both you and your doctor to handle questions and provide guidance about your care. Many transplant teams encourage patients to return to the transplant center annually, at least for the first few years, for follow-up care.

Find out whether the transplant center will keep your local doctor updated on your progress. Ask if you and your doctor will receive a survivorship care plan with written instructions about follow-up care. Both you and your doctor should feel comfortable contacting your transplant center directly to discuss questions and concerns.

Guidelines for long-term follow-up care have been developed by the American Society for Blood and Marrow Transplantation, the Center for International Blood & Marrow Transplant Research and the European Society for Blood and Marrow Transplantation. You can access these guidelines through the BMT InfoNet website at bmtinfonet.org/long-term-health-guidelines or by phoning 888-597-7674.

The Bottom Line

Happily, there are many excellent transplant programs that provide top-quality medical care. For most patients, no one program will clearly be superior. Rather, you and your doctor will be able to choose among many excellent, highly qualified transplant programs.

Keep in mind that you and your family are important members of the transplant team. It's important that you feel comfortable working with the staff at the center where you'll be treated. Together with your doctor, you should be able to identify the programs that best suit your family's medical, financial and emotional needs.

To learn more about transplant centers in the U.S go to our website at:

bmtinfonet.org/transplantcenters

Chapter Four

INSURANCE AND FUNDRAISING

Our insurance company said a transplant was experimental and would not approve it. During an unbelievably stressful week, we contacted an attorney, looked into private pay options and asked the hospital how they could help. I don't know whether it was the letters from our transplant center and our attorney, or calls from us and my employer that did it, but a week later they changed their mind and agreed to pay for the transplant.

Julie Brodeur, mother of a 5-year transplant survivor

Most transplant centers are skilled at providing insurers with the documentation they need to authorize coverage of an autologous transplant. Fortunately, most patients have no difficulty persuading their insurer to pay for their treatment.

However, if you have difficulty with your insurance company, read on. The information in this section will help you understand how insurance companies make decisions, how you can appeal those decisions, when to enlist the help of an experienced attorney and what other funding options exist.

An autologous transplant is a very expensive medical procedure. Depending on the transplant center, the length of time you must be hospitalized and complications that arise, the treatment can cost hundreds of thousands of dollars. It's therefore not surprising that insurance providers are cautious when reviewing requests to approve this treatment.

The best way to minimize insurance problems is to start early. Since life gets more hectic if an insurance denial comes at the last minute, it's important that you and the transplant team begin interacting with the insurance company early in the transplant process.

Pre-Approval for Treatment

As soon as possible, the transplant center will ask your insurer to pre-approve the treatment. It may take several weeks to get an answer from the insurance company. If you're covered by Medicare, you will not receive approval in advance. Medicare approves payment after treatment is completed.

The transplant center should set a target date for starting your treatment and communicate that date to the insurer when they seek pre-approval. This gives the insurer a deadline by which it must decide whether to pay for the treatment.

Most transplant centers send an information package to the insurer that includes a letter from the treating physician, as well as studies and articles supporting the recommended procedure. It's important that insurers get this information early on, and that it is complete and up-to-date. The letter from your transplant doctor should stress that the treatment is the best available therapy for you, is safe and effective and is widely accepted by the medical community. Articles and letters of support that explain why your transplant plan is appropriate should be current.

If Insurance Coverage is Denied

If your insurance company denies coverage of your medical treatment, it may be possible to reverse that decision. At some transplant centers, the transplant team will appeal the denial of coverage for you. The appeal process may require your transplant physician to call the reviewing physician at the insurance company. Most questions can be resolved with a physician-to-physician conversation.

If you must file an appeal on your own, it's wise to consult an attorney who is experienced in this field of law to determine whether or not you may be able to reverse a denial of coverage. Your letter of appeal should not be drafted by the attorney who helped you with your

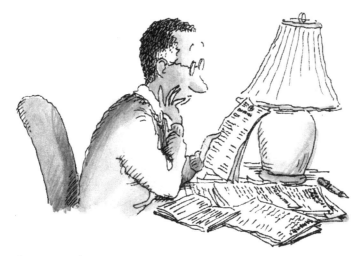

house closing or divorce. You need an attorney who is just as experienced in this field of law as your doctor is in this field of medicine.

Most insurance plans are governed by ERISA, a federal law that requires you to take steps within certain time frames. You are usually required to appeal a denial of coverage within 60 days or you lose all further rights of appeal.

What you put in the letter of appeal will determine your rights later should you have to go to court. You and your doctor should include *all* evidence supporting transplant as the appropriate therapy for you when you file the appeal. If you later must go to court to challenge the decision, the issue will be whether or not the insurer made an appropriate decision in light of the evidence it previously received from your doctor. You may not be able to offer additional evidence later at trial.

If insurance does not cover all of your transplant expenses, there are some other options to consider.

Viatical Settlements and Accelerated Life Insurance Benefits

Life insurance was once considered a source of funds only after a person died. However, two options are available for some owners of life insurance who are terminally or chronically ill — viatical settlements and accelerated life insurance benefits. Both provide cash benefits while the policyholder is still alive.

Viatical Settlements

Viatical settlements appeared in the 1980s in reaction to the AIDS crisis. Brokers offered to purchase life insurance policies at a discount from terminally ill patients. They would then sell them to a viatical settlement provider who made a cash payment to the patient. Patients were free to use the money for medical expenses, or any other purpose.

Soon an industry arose with good and bad results. Patients who truly needed cash had a new source of funds. However, some received far less than the true value of their policy.

To ensure that vulnerable patients are protected, many states now require viatical settlement providers to be licensed. If you are considering a viatical settlement, check with your state Department of Insurance to be sure the viatical firm is licensed. You can also check whether it is licensed to practice in states with strong consumer protection regulations on viatical settlements — New York, Washington or Florida.

Accelerated Benefits

Many life insurance policies have a specific accelerated benefits option. Some policies offer up to 75 percent of your benefit now, with the balance reserved as a true death benefit for your heirs. There is usually a fee charged for taking an accelerated benefit.

The advantages of taking accelerated benefits rather than selling a policy to a viatical settlement provider are two-fold: it is often less costly to take accelerated benefits, and you have the advantage of working with someone you know and trust. A disadvantage is that the insurance company may restrict the amount of benefits you can accelerate or put restrictions on how you use the funds.

Is It Right for Me?

If you are considering a viatical settlement or accelerating your life insurance benefits, here are some questions to think about:

1. Is there really a need for the money?

    Funds you withdraw now will not be available to pay for

expenses they were originally intended to cover such as educa-
tion and living expenses of your survivors. Examine why you
want the funds and consider if there are other options for securing necessary cash.

2. How will a viatical settlement or receipt of accelerated benefits
affect your overall financial picture?

The cash you receive from a viatical settlement or accelerated
benefits may affect your entitlement to public benefits, treatment of estate taxes and how your creditors view you. Check
with a social worker or benefits counselor to determine the
settlement's effect on benefits such as disability or Medicaid.
Speak with your accountant or attorney to determine what the
tax and estate consequences will be.

3. Does your insurance policy provide accelerated benefits?

Before entering into a viatical settlement, check to see if your life
insurance plan offers an accelerated benefits option. Accelerated
benefits can be cheaper and easier than a viatical settlement because it is already part of your policy.

4. Get the best deal.

Some viatical settlements offer the patient as little as 30 percent
of the total value of the life insurance policy. On a $300,000 life
insurance policy, that would be $90,000 to you and $210,000 to
the settlement provider. Shop around for the best deal. Consult
with a neutral, reputable financial advisor to help you understand the pros and cons of each plan you are considering.

Other Fundraising Options

Depending on your disease and income, you may be eligible for
financial support from one of the following organizations that help
autologous transplant patients:

Blood & Marrow Transplant Information Network
bmtinfonet.org
888-597-7674

The Bone Marrow Foundation
bonemarrow.org
800-365-1336

The Leukemia & Lymphoma Society
lls.org
800-955-4572

Lymphoma Research Foundation
lymphoma.org
800-500-9976

For a list of other groups that may help, go to BMT InfoNet's online Resource Directory at bmtinfonet.org/resource-directory or phone 888-597-7674.

If family members and friends are looking for a way to help you, ask them to hold a fundraiser for you. The following organizations help transplant patients organize fundraisers and manage the funds:

Help Hope Live
helphopelive.org
800-642-8399

National Foundation for Transplants
https://transplants.org
800-489-3863

Children's Organ Transplant Association
cota.org
800-366-2682

Online fundraising platforms like GoFundMe.com can be helpful in raising funds to cover transplant expenses.

To learn more, go to our website at:

bmtinfonet.org/insurance-and-financial-issues

Chapter Five

EMOTIONAL CHALLENGES

There weren't any support groups for transplant patients in my area. If there had been a support group, I would have attended, because when they first tell you about the transplant and you start reading up on the subject, it can scare the heck out of you.

Dwight Gambral, 13-year transplant survivor

Autologous transplantation provides hope for many patients diagnosed with diseases that were once thought incurable. This hope sustains patients and their families through the difficult period of treatment and recovery. Nonetheless, contemplating an autologous transplant, undergoing the procedure and coping with the recovery process can be a trying experience for patients and their family.

This chapter will discuss fears and emotions that are common during transplant. Throughout the chapter you will find quotations from people who have been through transplant and have offered to share their insights.

Coping with the News

When you learn that you need an autologous transplant, the news can be devastating. You may have not yet come to grips with the fact that you're suffering from a life-threatening disease. Deciding whether to undergo a transplant can increase the emotional turmoil. Sometimes the decision must be made quickly to provide the greatest likelihood of success, adding more stress to an already difficult situation.

The sheer volume of information can be overwhelming. If you are unfamiliar with medical jargon, that may make it difficult for you to understand doctors' explanations. You may find it hard to absorb new information while you are still struggling with so many other details about your disease. You may need to ask the same question many times before you understand the answer.

Little of the information you hear will sound like good news. What most people want to hear is that the transplant will be a quick, painless, risk-free procedure. More importantly, they want assurance that it will cure them of their disease and provide them with many extra years of life. Unfortunately, no such assurances can be given. You can only be promised the chance for a future.

Fear that more unsettling news is forthcoming stops many patients from asking questions. As much as they may want answers, some opt to cope with uncertainty rather than open themselves up to more disturbing information.

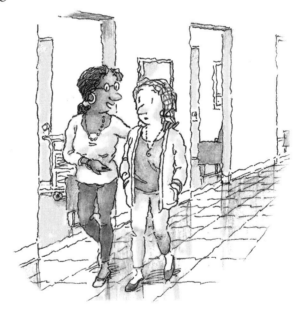

Getting Information

Your doctors will strive hard to give you a complete and honest description of the transplant experience. They want you to be fully informed about possible risks before undergoing the procedure. In doing so, however, doctors sometimes confuse and overwhelm patients. They may assume that you are familiar with medical terms like catheters, aspirates and biopsies. Often that is not the case. As one patient put it, "doctors talk medical, patients talk human."

Don't be embarrassed to ask your doctor to repeat something or re-state it in words you can understand. Sometimes, asking one of the nurses to explain what the doctor means will help you better under-stand the message. Keep asking questions until you're satisfied with the answer, regardless of how many times it takes.

Write down and prioritize any questions you have before visiting your doctor. Having a family member or friend accompany you to the visit can help you recall important details afterwards. Some pa-tients find that recording their initial discussion with the transplant team helps answer questions later. Others find that keeping an ongo-ing file with brochures, handouts, personal notes and resource infor-mation to refer to throughout the process helps.

> "Your mind is going to explode with all the things you have
> to remember or want to ask. Write down the questions
> you want to ask as well as the doctor's answers to your
> questions. If you don't get a straight answer or don't un-
> derstand the answer, ask again until it is clear."

> "It's important to make sure that the doctor talks with you
> about the items on YOUR agenda, not just his. You need
> to be assertive. My 23-year-old daughter, for example,
> wanted to talk about infertility and options for having a
> child after the transplant. The doctors wanted to brush
> that issue aside."

Putting Things into Perspective

For many patients, the list of possible complications is frightening and overwhelming. Ask your doctor to help you put them into per-spective. Don't assume that the risk of severe organ damage, for ex-ample, is as great as the risk of temporary hair loss or mouth sores. It's not!

You may find it helpful to group the possible complications into three categories:

- those that will definitely occur
- those that often occur
- those that rarely occur

This can help ease your worries about complications that are unlikely to happen.

Doctors sometimes forget to mention that pain relief will be provided when needed. Thus, when patients hear about possible complications, they worry that they'll be in terrible pain. There are many effective pain medications available to relieve any discomfort that might occur. Your transplant team will carefully monitor you for pain, and provide pain medication as needed. (For more about pain see Chapter Ten, Relieving Pain.)

Setting Goals

The time spent undergoing and recovering from a transplant can seem endless. Patients seldom make daily progress by leaps and bounds. Each day will bring a small step forward, maybe a little backsliding or no change at all. This slow pace of progress can discourage patients (and their loved ones) who want to get well and put this chapter of their life behind them.

Ask the doctors and nurses to help you set realistic goals, and to tell you each time progress is made, no matter how small. Any progress or positive news can boost your spirits.

> "Progress can be so very slow. I found it was helpful to keep charts so that I could see that progress was being made. Drinking an ounce of water an hour adds up to a lot of fluid by the end of the day. Walking three feet today and increasing it by two feet each day is a lot by the end of the week."

It helps to take one day at a time rather than worry about what will happen in five days or five years.

Loss of Control

> "In the beginning, I was a very angry patient. I was very bitter and scared. Anger was my way of coping."

An autologous transplant can be a physically debilitating experience. You may be in a fragile state of health for several weeks following the transplant, and may feel weak and helpless. Walking without assistance, focusing on a book or television show, following the thread of a conversation or even sitting up in bed may require more energy you have to spare.

If you are used to being in charge, taking care of yourself or being the person upon whom others depend, you may find your physical weakness discouraging. The loss of control frightens and angers some patients, and their anger is sometimes directed at medical personnel or loved ones.

Patients often react angrily to people who try to dictate, rather than tactfully encourage them to do things they would rather not do. Giving the patient a chance to exert some control over his or her care may reduce feelings of helplessness and anger.

Feelings of Isolation

The special precautions taken to protect against infection while your immune system is recovering may make you feel lonely and isolated. Transplant patients crave a normal environment where they're not the center of attention, where they can interact freely with family and friends and where they can think about something other than their disease and treatment.

While you are hospitalized or staying in a facility away from home, decorating your room with things that are special to you can help make you feel less detached from normal life. Bringing in your own bed clothes and other personal belongings can make the room seem homier.

When family and friends call or visit, they should talk about the world outside. Positive, upbeat stories about family members and friends, descriptions of stores or museums visited, plays or movies that they've seen, the latest gossip from work or school — anything that brings the outside world to you — can make you feel less isolated and cut off from normal life.

Stressful Side Effects

Some side effects of high-dose chemotherapy or radiation can be stressful. Temporary hair loss may change your self-image and make you feel embarrassed to be seen by family or friends. Wearing a head scarf or hat may make you feel less conspicuous and, for some, is more comfortable than a wig.

Meals, too, can be stressful. Mouth sores, a common side effect of treatment, can make eating uncomfortable. Some of the drugs you receive may temporarily alter the taste of foods. (For more on eating difficulties see Chapter Nine, Nutrition.)

The large quantity of medications you will need to take orally each day can be daunting and you may have difficulty trying to force down the pills. The tests that monitor your physical condition, while not painful, can be stressful.

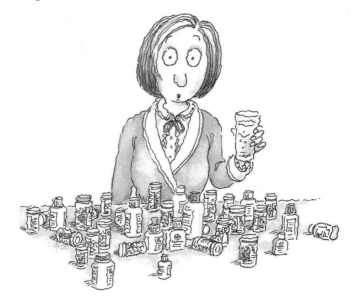

In some cases, it is possible to reduce the physical discomfort associated with a procedure and thus reduce stress. Lightly sedating a patient prior to a bone marrow biopsy, for example, can make the procedure more comfortable. Do not be reluctant to ask for pre-medication or other pain relief if you're worried about discomfort.

Family members should take an assertive role in telling doctors and nurses about any pain you have. The medical team needs to know if you are likely to request relief as soon as pain begins or only after the discomfort is really intense. The speed with which they respond to your call for help can be influenced by this important information. (For more about pain relief see Chapter Ten, Relieving Pain.)

Managing Anxiety

Anxiety and distress are a normal, expected part of the transplant experience. Patients who become very anxious or agitated are not weak or losing their mind. They're reacting in a very normal way to a very stressful experience.

"During my transplant I was very depressed. My dad asked a co-worker, who had a transplant five years earlier, to visit me and share what he had been through. He said my feelings were acceptable, that he had been depressed, too, but now he's better and working full-time. I could look at him and see that he was a normal person. That helped me more than anything."

> It's important to be honest with your own feelings. If you need help dealing with what you are about to face, seek it. This is not a sign of weakness. Sometimes, talking with someone who's been through the situation helps you separate, evaluate and move in a healthier direction.

You may benefit from talking with a psychiatrist, psychologist or social worker. If your physician does not volunteer these helpful services to you, ask for them.

Psychiatrists often help patients manage anxiety with sedatives and anti-depressant medications. Short-term use of these drugs by transplant patients is common, and does not lead to long-term drug dependency.

Insomnia

Transplant patients often have insomnia — difficulty falling or staying asleep. Deprived of sleep, you can quickly become exhausted, unfocused and extremely irritable, making it even harder to cope with daytime stresses. Medications are available to counteract insomnia. There's no need to put up with sleepless nights and the stress they produce. Like all medications, however, they may cause side effects that you should discuss with your transplant doctor.

> "Right before the transplant I had a lot of trouble sleeping. The whole thing was such a shock. Eventually a friend of mine who is a pediatrician suggested I get a prescription for sleeping pills. They really helped and they weren't addictive."

> "I had trouble sleeping when going through my transplant, and still do sometimes. I find that active relaxation helps. Rather than laying awake, I get up and do some exercises — a few leg lifts or sit ups. It helps me relax and get back to sleep."

Keeping in Touch with Friends

Throughout much of your treatment and recovery, you may be too weak to visit with guests or even accept phone calls. Nonetheless, it helps to know that family members, friends and co-workers are concerned about your progress. Cards and words of encouragement from family and friends can mean a lot to a patient who is feeling isolated.

> "My family and friends put together an album for me when I was in the hospital, and everyone contributed something. There were pictures and all sorts of silly things — it was wonderful. Another friend, who is a professional photographer, gathered everyone in the park, took their picture and blew it up. I'm talking poster-size. It included everyone — my family, my friends, my co-workers — everyone. I loved it."

> "I arranged for my wife to hear messages left by well-wishers on our answering machine. It cheered her to know that so many people were thinking of her, and it eliminated the problem of having the phone ring when she wasn't up to taking calls."

If you have access to the internet, websites like CaringBridge.org are a great way to keep in touch with family and friends. You, or a family member, can create a personal web page to post daily updates about your progress for people to read. Visitors to your site can leave news about what's going on in their life as well as words of encouragement for you. Facebook and personal blogs are another way to keep family and friends up-to-date on what is happening.

Sometimes people are afraid to intrude and therefore do not call or write. If you are a friend or family member who is concerned about intruding, check first with a close family member. More often than not, your expression of concern will boost the patient's spirits.

Other gestures like helping with family household chores, caring for the patient's children, providing an evening off for the patient's care-giver or filling in for the patient until he or she returns to work will also be greatly appreciated.

> "My co-workers cut my grass, brought meals and cleaned my house. During a heat wave, my church installed an air conditioner in my husband's room. Accepting this help was uplifting. I felt like I wasn't alone."

> "One thing that friends and co-workers did that did NOT help was tell me stories about people with cancer who didn't make it. I didn't really need to hear that and sometimes that can still set me off. Instead of saying, 'Please don't share any more with me,' or, 'I'd prefer not to hear this', I'd just stand there and listen. That was stupid. In retrospect, I should have just politely cut it off."

Family members, friends and co-workers sometimes have difficulty re-establishing a relationship with the patient after transplant. You may look different. You may have lost weight, be wearing a face mask to protect against infection, look physically drained or have no hair. Because you will have been out of circulation for several weeks, you will not have shared as many experiences with family members or friends as usual. Visitors can feel awkward as they grope for an appropriate topic of conversation, and this awkwardness can discourage some people from calling or visiting.

> "I had one friend who was so afraid to come near me that when she would visit, she'd drive up to the front of the house, beep her horn, wave to me and then drive off. That really hurt. Others would come right into my house, help wash and feed me — they were wonderful. They will always be my dearest and closest friends."

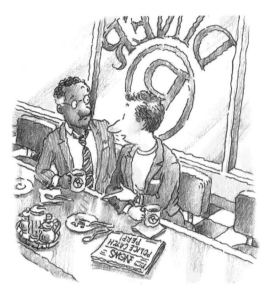

Friends and family members can overcome some of this post-transplant awkwardness by not losing touch with the patient while he or she is undergoing treatment. Sharing normal life experiences with the patient either during a visit, by a note or with a phone call can make re-establishing relationships after a transplant easier.

> "My friend Roz was really great. She'd call and say, 'How are you?' and then would start talking about all the things we used to talk about before the transplant. She wouldn't avoid the subject of the transplant, but she treated me just like she did before."

Often, friends will be unsure about how and when to re-establish a normal relationship with you, and will look for a cue from you before making a move. Ask friends to help with a small task such as picking up a prescription from the drug store, taking your child to a school event or returning a purchased item to a department store. This will signal your friends that you welcome their companionship.

Friends can help ease the transition back to normal life by inviting you to places or events that do not pose health risks. Even though physical changes, such as hair loss, may make you feel conspicuous, most patients have a strong desire to get back into the normal flow of life and appreciate the invitation.

Many Months Beyond Transplant

Although memories of the transplant experience dim with time, it may take many months before you can get through a single day without reflecting on the transplant experience. Innocent remarks or events totally unrelated to the transplant may stir up unpleasant memories, leaving you feeling shaken.

> "I used to get flashbacks for about a year after my transplant. I remember walking down the aisle of a grocery store, and I'd remember something about the transplant and get a big hit of adrenaline. But that pretty much ended when I made a conscious decision to stop worrying about relapse and the transplant."

During the first year after a transplant, some survivors find it hard to make long-term plans or commitments.

> "In the beginning, fear of relapse definitely affected my ability to make long-term commitments. I wouldn't start new projects or even pick out new clothes. I don't think I'll ever put it totally behind me, but I don't dwell on it anymore."

Many people who have been through transplant find the experience difficult to talk about. They prefer to forget about the past and go on with their life.

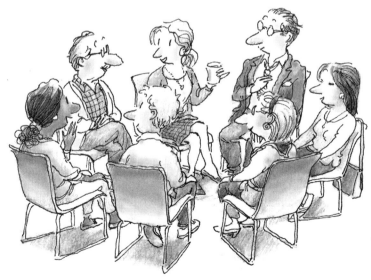

Others want an outlet to talk about the transplant. Support groups are helpful for some survivors, while others prefer to talk one-on-one with counselors, other transplant survivors, a family member or a friend.

> "The support group taught me how to talk about life's most difficult problems. The people in the group share the bond of an incredibly traumatic journey, and we're not afraid to help each other."

There are chat rooms and discussion lists on the internet where patients and survivors can communicate with each other. You can find links to these on BMT InfoNet's website at bmtinfonet.org/emotional-challenges or by phoning 888-597-7674.

Despite the emotional ups and downs, life after transplant can be very special. Survivors no longer take the future for granted and often enjoy life more fully.

> "Each day is special for me. When I get up in the morning I look at the grass and trees and marvel at how beautiful everything is. For me, the transplant was like starting over again. It gave me a whole new life."

To learn more, go to our website at:

bmtinfonet.org/emotional-challenges

Chapter Six

WHEN YOUR CHILD NEEDS A TRANSPLANT

It was like a whirlwind, a dream. One day our child was a normal 15-year-old boy who would live to be 80. The next day we were staring at blackboard diagrams about transplants, and hearing doctors tell us our son might die. It wasn't real. We didn't understand. All we could do was hug each other and cry.

Lorraine Boldt, mother of 11-year transplant survivor

"Your child needs a transplant" are some of the most difficult words a parent can hear. The uncertainty, feeling of helplessness and stress associated with deciding whether to proceed to transplant affects the entire family.

Young children may demonstrate rebellious or babyish behavior. Teens may express anger toward loved ones, engage in risky behavior or attempt to shut parents out. Young siblings may worry that they caused the child's disease or resent the extra attention the sick sibling receives. Stress in marital relationships may intensify as everyone tries to cope with the difficult situation.

One thing is true: a transplant is a family affair. Acknowledging that everyone feels scared, but that everyone is working hard to make your child well, can help your family pull together to face the challenges ahead.

Through everything, remember this: thousands of children have been through a transplant and are now living normal, healthy lives.

Deciding to Have a Transplant

Deciding whether to proceed with a transplant is a difficult decision for families. The odds of success must be weighed against the certainty that the transplant will be a lengthy, rigorous procedure. Sometimes there is no clear-cut right choice, and you and your child can feel frustrated about having to choose between several unpleasant options.

Getting easy-to-understand information about a transplant is not always easy. Some transplant centers provide only oral explanations of what to expect, while others provide written materials, such as this book. The information you receive can be overwhelming. It helps to have more than one adult present during meetings with medical personnel and to keep notes.

Sometimes parents receive conflicting information from their referring physician and the transplant team. The doctors may quote different survival rates or disagree about the timing of the transplant. Sometimes, parents do not learn about all the complications associated with a transplant until they meet with the transplant team.

> "The first conference with the transplant team was the most depressing experience of my life — worse than when my daughter was diagnosed. The doctor that referred us to the transplant center never told us about the possible side effects. I was terrified. I just wanted to grab my child and run."

Don't be shy about asking questions. Bring a list of questions to your meeting with doctors and keep asking until you feel you have enough information to make a decision. It is the medical team's job to make sure all questions are answered, no matter how long or how many repetitions it takes.

Many parents find it helpful to talk to other parents whose child went through a transplant. BMT InfoNet's Caring Connections program can put you in contact with other parents. You can access this service online at bmtinfonet.org/caring-connection or by phone

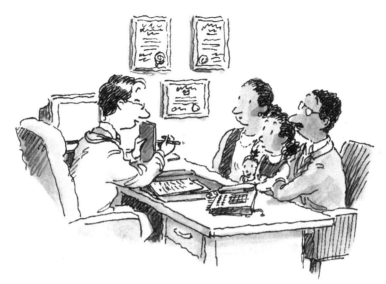

at 888-597-7674. Keep in mind, however, that despite their similarities, no two families' experiences will be exactly alike.

Let your child ask questions as well. It is important to involve your child in the decision-making process and secure his or her cooperation and trust.

In most states, if your child is under age 14, you are responsible for making the final decision about whether to proceed with a transplant. Nonetheless, it is the child who must live with the consequences and this can create internal turmoil for parents.

> "I knew it was a do or die situation but I kept asking myself, 'Do I really have the right to decide his life? I want to keep him with me as long as possible. Am I deciding what's best for me or for him?' "

Disagreements between parents, or between parents and children, about the wisdom of proceeding with a transplant are common.

> "We had just gotten our son back to the point where he seemed happy and healthy and now they were proposing a transplant. I kept thinking, 'Why take him back to ground zero? Why can't we leave him alone?' "

It's important to listen to each other carefully and to respect each other's concerns as much as your own.

Preparing Siblings

Once you've decided to proceed with a transplant, the treatment should be carefully explained to siblings. Involving siblings in discussions about your child's disease and treatment early on can help unite the family.

> "We decided our 12-year-old son and his brother would be told honestly about what was happening, and both would participate in decision-making as much as their age and maturity allowed. Although this placed a burden of maturity on both sons, they rose to meet it and our family drew closer, frequently drawing support from each other."

Families who involve siblings in discussions about the child's care and treatment often have fewer problems later on with jealousy or anger. Be completely honest with both the child and siblings from the start so there are no surprises down the road and no feelings that they've been lied to.

Questions Children Ask

Children's questions and concerns about the transplant vary depending on their age. Younger children focus on immediate problems like how much it will hurt, whether they will be separated from their parents and when they can return to school. They may ask when their hair will grow back and whether they'll vomit a lot.

If they've received prior treatment for their disease, they may worry

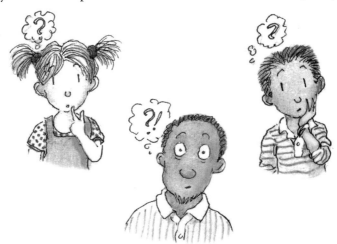

about whether they will have chemotherapy again. After acquiring a basic understanding of the procedure, younger children tend to rely on their parents to decide what's best.

Teens, on the other hand, take a much more active role in the decision-making process. They tend to be very concerned about self-image and focus on issues like losing their hair and fitting back in with their peers once the transplant is over.

The possibility of infertility after transplant can be distressing for an adolescent. Sexual identity and activity are important to teens. Many don't understand the distinction between being fertile and being sexually active. It helps to tell them that many adults are infertile, yet lead a normal sex life. It's also important to help them distinguish between childbearing and child-rearing.

Preparing for Medical Procedures

Preparing your child for each new medication or medical procedure is important. Your child needs to know what will be done, what the equipment will look like and how he or she will feel. Tell your child about the medication or procedure far enough in advance to allow for questions, but not so far in advance that there's time to brood about it.

Advance preparation is even required before the administration of drugs designed to ease pain or sedate your child.

> "The first time my child was given Demerol® he became almost violent. He wasn't prepared for the fact that he'd feel groggy and it frightened him. After that, I always made sure he knew in advance how the drugs would make him feel."

It helps to let your child rehearse medical procedures in advance, or to practice the procedure on dolls or adults. Break the procedure into small steps, moving on to the next step only after your child's anxiety about the first step has been relieved.

You can be an important advocate for your child, particularly when it comes to securing pain relief or minimizing the discomfort associated with medical procedures. Some centers, for example, administer seda-

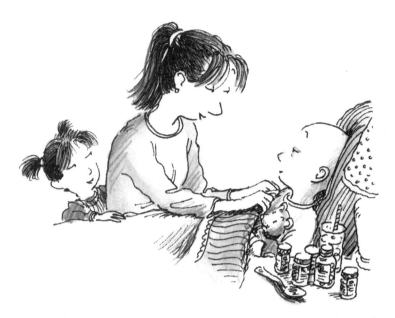

tives to children in advance of a bone marrow aspirate, while others do not. Don't hesitate to ask for pain medication if your child has difficulty with a procedure.

Coping with Anxiety

Once preparations for the transplant have been finalized, families can feel uneasy. Everyone will be anxious, and you may agonize over the wisdom of proceeding with this treatment.

> "You have to learn to have confidence in your ability to make decisions, and believe you made the best choice under the circumstance. Don't panic about what may happen, and don't fret about what has happened. It can't be changed. Just take one day at a time."

For most children, the transplant will be the hardest challenge they've ever faced. Younger children may fear that they are to blame for the disease and treatment. They may think they were somehow bad and are now being punished. Young siblings may also fear that they somehow caused the problem.

It's important to encourage children of all ages to discuss their feelings openly so their concerns can be addressed. Find out what your child is thinking. Don't assume that if he or she doesn't talk about the illness or transplant, there's no problem.

Some children express their anxieties by behavioral changes such as belligerence, depression or poor performance in school. Let them know that you understand they're unhappy, frightened and confused, and that you're unhappy, too. Assure them that everyone will work hard to make your child well again.

Sometimes children will more openly discuss their feelings with someone other than their parents. This is particularly true of pre-adolescents and adolescents who are fearful of hurting their parents' feelings or causing them distress. Adolescents who are coping with typical teen desires for independence may be especially reluctant to let down their guard in the presence of parents.

It's important to allow children to discuss their feelings with whomever they feel most comfortable. You can seek the help of nurses, psychologists or other counselors to encourage your child to talk about his or her concerns.

Life During Transplant

Although a transplant is anything but routine, it is important to maintain as much of your child's normal home routine as possible. Bringing favorite clothes, pictures and toys to the hospital helps maintain a sense of normalcy.

Arrange for calls, letters and/or visits from your child's classmates, favorite teacher, church members or a hometown doctor with whom your child feels comfortable. Some families make videos of family and friends that the child can view while in the hospital.

Boredom in the hospital can be a big issue for children. Bringing favorite toys and games from home helps to ease the boredom. Planning diversions and activities for teens is especially important.

> "My son, who was 15 years old, was transplanted at a children's hospital. Although they had lots of activities planned, they were usually geared toward younger kids, not teens."

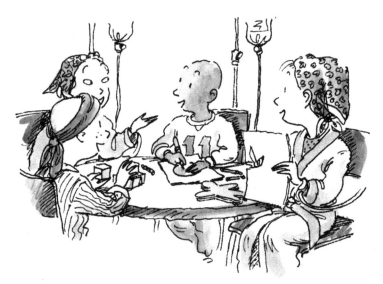

Loss of Control

Despite everyone's best efforts, the hospitalization will be a very stressful time for you and your child alike. Your child may feel overwhelmed by the daily tests, medical procedures and many medications.

Children of all ages, and teens in particular, feel overwhelmed by all the rules and bosses, and can become angry over the loss of personal control. This can manifest itself in a variety of ways.

Some become angry or belligerent, refusing to cooperate with parents or the medical staff. Others will cry for no apparent reason and may be unable to explain what is making them sad.

Some children refuse to eat or play. Others become depressed, listless or exhibit regressive or babyish behavior. They may be incapable of performing tasks they were previously able to do on their own.

Children spend a whole lot of time and energy growing up, seizing control over their lives and becoming more independent. When they undergo a transplant, they lose that independence and control, and that can make them angry or depressed.

Children don't feel the same urgency about routine medical procedures as parents do. It's important to let your child know that you understand that it's hard, and that feeling angry is normal and okay.

"I never said to my son, 'don't cry'. I encouraged him to talk about what was bothering him and to let it all out. If he really rebelled against doing something like mouth care, I wouldn't insist it be done that moment. We'd talk about it and usually it would get done without a fight five minutes later. Sometimes I'd suggest we do it a few minutes before the nurse came in so that he could feel like it was his decision and not her order that made it happen. He liked that feeling of control."

Children are as concerned about protecting their bodies and having control over their personal life as adults. Give your child the opportunity to say no or to make choices regarding daily care and activities whenever it's possible for you to honor that decision.

Setting up and sticking to a daily routine in the hospital is important for children. Ideally, the routine should include some safe time for your child each day during which no unpleasant tests, medications or staff interventions occur. One child's parents created a safe area for their daughter in the hospital room by bringing in a free-standing tent. When the child needed time alone, she would go into the tent to play.

Challenges for Parents

The time in the hospital can be challenging for parents. It's hard to watch your child undergo difficult medical procedures, particularly when you have so little control over his or her care.

"They kept saying that being there for my child was important but it never felt like I was doing enough."

It is important for you to pace yourself so that you don't become exhausted or ill. Taking a few minutes or hours off while social workers or visitors spend time with your child can be helpful. Some parents find that spending the night away from the hospital enables them to get a good night's rest and better cope with the next day's stresses. For other parents, remaining with the child overnight is less stressful.

"At first it was hard for me to leave my child each night, and I tried to get the hospital to change their policy.

But it became a haven for me — I could take a hot bath, watch television, sleep and have some time to myself."

"My mother and sister would sometimes stay with my son while I went to a nearby mall or got my hair done. Just getting outside, even for a few minutes, made a tremendous difference."

Children are very perceptive about their parents' feelings and can be frightened when they detect sadness or stress in their parents. Some children may feel guilty, thinking they caused their parents' sadness, and a desire to protect their parents can be a stumbling block to speaking frankly about their own concerns. Acknowledging that the hospitalization is scary for everyone and that you will work through the experience together is important.

"Every day my son would say, 'I love you. Thank you for being here with me. It makes it easier when I'm not feeling good.' He knew it was just as hard for me as it was for him."

Siblings' Care

Often siblings must be left in the care of friends or relatives while their brother or sister is undergoing a transplant. Removed from their home and normal routines, young children may view the separation from their parents as a punishment. It is important that siblings know that you don't want to be away from them, that the separation will be temporary and why it's not possible for them to be with you.

Set up a plan of routine contact between you and your child's siblings so they don't feel they are being ignored or aren't loved as much as the sick child.

"Every day I would call my daughter and write her a note. When I wrote, I would tell her what was happening with her brother, but when I called, I made sure we talked about her."

Marital Stress

It is not unusual for problems that previously existed in a marriage to be heightened during this time. Plans for a separation or divorce may get put on hold as a result of the transplant, with tensions between marital partners increasing. The additional stress may cause substance abuse.

Don't be embarrassed to seek help for these problems — you won't be the first. In general, it's best to make as few changes as possible in the home routine and keep lines of communication open during this difficult time.

Even parents who previously felt they had a good relationship can experience marital tensions. Often, one parent remains at the hospital with the child, while the spouse spends most of his or her time at home, continuing to work, taking care of the home and caring for the other children. Both may be thrust into roles they normally don't assume.

The caregiver at the hospital needs to deal with complicated medical issues, a child who is physically and emotionally exhausted and his or her own exhaustion and emotions. There's little or no break from the stress.

The spouse who remains home may assume more child care and household responsibilities, and must deal with his or her own fears as well as the emotional needs of the other children. He or she may feel left out or poorly informed about what's happening each day with the sick child.

Both parents will be under stress and need each other's support. However, both may be too exhausted or upset to understand how their spouse feels and what he or she needs. As one mother put it, "Stress like this will either make a marriage stronger or pull it apart."

> "I was at the hospital 24 hours a day. My husband was able
> to re-enter the world when he became overwhelmed, go
> to the office, pretend to live a normal life. When we
> came home, he wanted things to return to normal, but
> I was just starting to look back and process what we had
> been through. I was coping with the anger and fear I
> couldn't focus on in the hospital. I was extremely angry
> that he couldn't see things the way I did. One night I felt
> like our marriage was over. I told him he didn't under-
> stand where I'd been. He said, 'I've been there, too.'

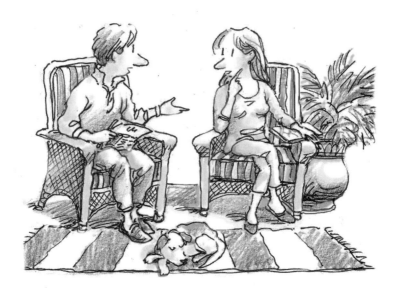

We went to therapy together and were able to address a lot of issues."

"I was a raving lunatic and my husband didn't understand why. I was dead tired and would have liked for him to pick up the slack. He couldn't do it. He was devastated when our child got sick — he'd never had to handle a catastrophe like this before. Sometimes, I just needed a big hug from him but he wasn't capable of it. I got mad and snippy with him when he wouldn't do little things like taking out the garbage without being asked. I started to resent him. I finally realized that if you have bad feelings, you have to talk about it, even if your husband isn't a talker. It takes work to keep a marriage together under these circumstances. It's not a piece of cake."

"It's important to respect each other's differences. I think men and women handle crises in different ways. My husband and I handled our fears differently. One way is not necessarily better than the other."

Going Home

Going home — the day that everyone waits for — can be a bittersweet experience. Although the hospitalization has ended, the recovery period is far from over. Medications must be administered several times daily, central lines must be cleaned and there will be daily, then weekly visits to the outpatient clinic to monitor progress. You will be on pins and needles watching for complications.

> "You think you'll get to go home and lead a normal life but it's not like that. Living at home with a child who has a weak immune system is scary. We constantly worried that my husband would bring home germs from work, and we carried disinfectant everywhere."

It is common for problems to develop that require your child to be re-admitted to the hospital for a short time. This can be alarming for you and your child alike.

> "You never know what will come up. Since we've come home, we've had many trips to the hospital. There's still a lot of home care for our daughter. Every time something goes wrong I feel guilty, thinking that something I did made my child worse. Wrong thoughts, I know, but we're only human."

Sometimes behavioral problems surface after transplant. Parents are in an awkward position. While in the hospital, your child may have received lots of cards, gifts, balloons and attention, and may expect it to continue when he or she returns home.

Frequently, friends and extended family fail to understand that the trauma continues long after your child returns home.

> "They think that once you walk out the door of the hospital, everything is behind you, and you should pick up life where you left off. It just doesn't work that way."

> "It would really drive me crazy when people would say, 'You must feel so lucky,' or 'You must be so grateful,' when I was feeling anything but lucky. While I was grateful to have witnessed a miracle, I was still really angry that our family had to go through all this."

The reunion of the siblings with the parent who spent time at the hospital with the transplant child is not always a smooth one.

"At first my three-year-old refused to talk to me. My daughter was left in my husband's care at home during my son's transplant. She talked with my husband and treated him like her parent but closed up to me. That hurt a lot. We found a therapist who helped us understand her fears and resentments, and work through them."

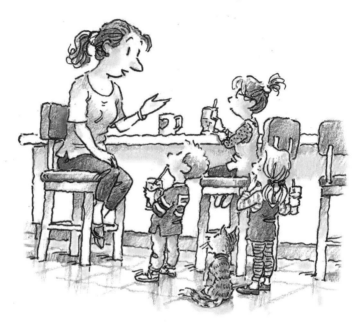

Siblings can become jealous about the extra attention the transplant survivor receives after returning home. They may express a desire to be sick so that you pay more attention to them. They can resent the fact that different rules apply to them than to the transplant child.

Some parents find that involving siblings in the routine caregiving can make them feel needed and important. Setting aside time for the parent and sibling to do something special together also helps.

"My four-year-old daughter was not pleased when my son came home from the hospital. There was a lot of whining, crying and naughtiness like biting. She directed her anger at me, not my son. I tried to find special things for her — like special times for her to be with her parents or special treats when we'd take my son to the clinic. That seemed to help."

"My five-year-old cried a lot. She kept asking, 'Why is my sister always sick? Why does she get extra attention?' I told her that I loved them equally, and I talked with her about what it was like when she was a little baby like her sister. I told her mommy was with her the whole time and paid lots of attention to her. I said, 'It's okay to be angry, but it's not your sister's fault — don't be angry with her.' I feel like I missed a good bit of my five-year-old because I was so preoccupied with the baby and her problems from birth. Now I try to make up the difference in healthy ways."

Getting Back to Normal

Getting back to normal will be a slow process. For many months after the transplant, both the transplant survivor and siblings may become anxious over symptoms of a common cold or other minor discomforts.

> Don't assume siblings' complaints of illness are a deliberate ploy to get your attention. Children often mimic symptoms of the illness unconsciously and truly believe they are ill.

"I went to my son's room one night when I heard him sniffling. 'This feels so familiar,' he said. 'I always used to get sick at night and you'd have to take me to the hospital.' When I assured him that he would be okay, he said, 'That sounds familiar, too.' "

"Our daughter was afraid to get sick after her brother's transplant. When she got the flu last week it was the first time that she was the sick one rather than her brother. He hovered over her, rubbed her back and brought her something to drink, trying to soothe her. They were both very concerned."

Don't ignore or trivialize a sibling's complaints of illness. Show your child you are as concerned about his or her well-being as you are about the child who has had a transplant.

Certain events that parents view as milestones can be very traumatic for a child. A two-year-old, for example, became very upset when his central venous catheter was removed. "We thought he'd be happy to get rid of it. Instead, he became very upset. It was like part of his body was being removed," said his mother.

Returning to school is a milestone that children are encouraged to look forward to, but it, too, can be a tremendous letdown. They may find their classmates are not anxiously awaiting their return. Their friends may have moved on to new interests and activities without them. Some children may be afraid to associate with a child who has been sick and now looks different.

It helps to prepare classmates in advance for your child's return. A nurse, doctor or social worker can visit the school, explain what has happened to your child and answer questions. Even with advance preparation, however, your child may find it difficult to fit back in. The Leukemia and Lymphoma Society offers a package of materials to help parents and teachers prepare children for the return of a classmate who has been ill.

Despite the difficulties, the transplant experience often brings families closer together:

> "My children still squabble a lot, but they're very concerned and protective of each other as well. It was rough while we went through it, but the good times have come now. My son made it, he's healthy and we all appreciate what it means to be alive."

To learn more, go to our website at:

bmtinfonet.org/talking-children-about-transplants

Chapter Seven

CONDITIONING/PREPARATIVE REGIMEN

The doctor spent thirty minutes telling me all the things that could go wrong. Suddenly I could hear no more. 'Stop,' I said emphatically. 'I know you have to give me all the statistics, but I am not a statistic. My name is Harvey Erlich and I have an attitude problem. I refuse to die. Now, I believe that I can make it, do you?'

Harvey Erlich, 3-year transplant survivor

The conditioning regimen (also called the preparative regimen) is the high-dose chemotherapy and/or radiation given to patients during the week before their transplant.

The conditioning regimen is designed to destroy as many diseased cells as possible without major damage to your organs and tissues. Drugs used in the conditioning regimen are sometimes the same as those used in standard chemotherapy to treat the disease. The dosages, however, are much higher and more effective in killing diseased cells.

The high-dose chemotherapy and radiation also destroy the stem cells in the bone marrow. Therefore, an infusion of stem cells is required to rescue you from the effects of the conditioning regimen, even if the disease being treated has not spread to the bone marrow.

High-Dose Chemotherapy

Most conditioning regimens include high-dose chemotherapy. The chemotherapy drugs are usually administered over a one-to-six day period through a catheter that has been placed in a large vein near the chest. Some chemotherapy drugs are administered intravenously or taken as a pill.

Total Body Irradiation (TBI)

Some conditioning regimens include total body irradiation (TBI). TBI is typically administered to patients in one or more sessions over a one-to-seven day period. When TBI is administered over several days it is called fractionated TBI. If it is broken up into several lower-dosage sessions in a single day it is called hyperfractionated TBI.

While you do not actually see or feel the radiation, you may still find TBI an unnerving experience. You must sit or lie still, sometimes in an awkward position, for 10 to 45 minutes while the radiation is administered. This can be difficult, particularly if you are nauseated. Some transplant centers use special stands or boxes to help patients remain immobile during TBI. These can be confining and make some patients feel anxious.

Pre-medication with sedatives can help reduce anxiety. Children are usually sedated before TBI sessions to minimize their movement, and very young children may even be given anesthesia.

It helps to visit the radiation center before TBI therapy begins in order to familiarize yourself with the equipment and to get your questions answered. Most centers provide patients with a simulation of TBI therapy, so they know in advance what to expect, and so that the health care team can assure that dosages and equipment measurements are correct.

Common Short-Term Side Effects

High-dose chemotherapy and TBI are toxic to normal tissues and organs as well as diseased cells. Nausea, vomiting, diarrhea, mouth sores and temporary hair loss almost always occur to varying degrees regardless of which conditioning regimen is used. Severe or long-term damage to organs and tissues occurs much less frequently.

As you read the following sections, keep in mind that the degree to which people experience side effects differs and no one experiences all possible side effects.

Nausea, Vomiting and Diarrhea

Nausea and vomiting are common following all conditioning regimens but can be controlled with medication.

Drugs called antiemetics are used to prevent and treat nausea. Antiemetics can cause side effects such as anxiety, drowsiness and restlessness. Occasionally, muscle tightness, uncontrolled eye movement or shakiness can occur. These drug reactions can be frightening, but are usually less serious than they appear. Lowering the dosage of the antiemetic or administering an antihistamine usually reduces or eliminates the problem.

> Patients are often overwhelmed by the list of possible side effects from the conditioning regimen. **Keep in mind that most side effects are temporary and completely reversible, and that severe or long-term organ damage is the exception rather than the rule.** Discomfort associated with side effects can usually be prevented or relieved with medication.

Diarrhea following the conditioning regimen is also common. Antidiarrheal drugs can help control muscle contractions and diarrhea.

Mouth, Throat, Skin and Hair

High-dose chemotherapy and radiation target rapidly dividing cells, such as cancer cells. However, some normal cells also divide rapidly such as those that line the mouth, throat and gut, as well as hair and skin cells. These cells can be temporarily damaged by high-dose chemotherapy or radiation.

Mouth sores (mucositis) and throat sores (stomatitis) typically appear four-to-eight days following the conditioning regimen. Topical anesthetics, such as Lidocaine® or Dyclone®, or narcotics given intravenously, such as morphine, are used to relieve this discomfort. Frequently brushing your teeth and gums with a soft brush, and rinsing with a saline solution helps prevent mouth infections.

A drug called palifermin (Kepivance®) may lessen the severity and duration of mucositis. There are also rinses that can help reduce the discomfort caused by mouth sores.

Mucositis may make eating difficult or impossible. You may be fed intravenously until the discomfort ends. Intravenous feeding is also used if your stomach is unable to absorb sufficient nutrients as a result of temporary irritation caused by the conditioning regimen. Antacids may help to reduce stomach irritation. (For more on eating difficulties after transplant, see Chapter Nine, Nutrition.)

Temporary hair loss (alopecia) occurs following the conditioning regimen. Hair loss changes a patient's appearance and for some is very distressing. Scarves, hats or wigs can be used until the hair grows back. Some patients prefer to shave their heads or cut their hair very short before hair loss begins. Hair normally grows back within three-to-six months following the transplant. Sometimes the amount of curl or thickness of the new hair will differ from your hair before transplant. In rare cases, hair loss is permanent.

Skin rash is common following some of the conditioning regimens that include TBI, busulfan, etoposide, carmustine or thiotepa. Less often, dark spots on the skin, called hyperpigmentation, occur. Hyperpigmentation is most obvious in the creases of the skin and on fingernails and toenails. It is seen most often in people with darker skin. The spots usually fade in one-to-three months.

Bladder Irritation (hemorrhagic cystitis)
Bladder irritation, which can cause bloody or painful urination, sometimes occurs following the conditioning regimen, particularly those that include cyclophosphamide (Cytoxan®) or ifosfamide. Increasing the rate of intravenous fluids, using a catheter to irrigate the bladder or administering a drug called mesna (Mesnex®) are techniques commonly used to prevent or treat this problem.

Liver
Liver blood test abnormalities occur in approximately 50 percent of patients following the conditioning regimen, but only a few will actually develop liver damage. You may experience jaundice (yellowing of the skin), significant weight gain due to fluid retention and abnormal levels of liver enzymes and bilirubin (a pigment produced during the break up of red blood cells) in the blood. Resting the liver

and avoiding medications that aggravate the condition are the usual treatments until the liver heals itself.

Sinusoidal Obstruction Syndrome (SOS)

Sinusoidal obstruction syndrome (SOS), previously known as veno-occlusive disease (VOD), is a potentially serious liver problem caused by high-dose chemotherapy and/or TBI. The blood vessels that carry blood through the liver become swollen and blocked. Without a blood supply, the liver cannot remove toxins, drugs and other waste products from the bloodstream. Fluids build up in the liver causing swelling and tenderness. The kidneys may retain excess water and salt, causing swelling in the legs, arms and abdomen.

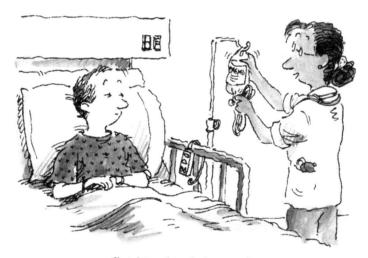

In severe cases, excess fluid in the abdominal cavity puts pressure on the lungs making it difficult to breathe. Toxins that are not processed out of the blood by the liver may affect how the brain functions and cause confusion, although confusion is a symptom of other, less serious problems as well.

In most cases, SOS is mild or moderate and the liver damage is reversible. SOS was once very difficult to treat, but a drug called defibrotide (Defitelio®) is now available to treat this complication.

Lungs and Heart

Breathing irregularities can occur following the conditioning regimen. Some patients develop pneumonia during the first four weeks after transplant. In most cases, injury to the lungs is mild and temporary, but some patients do experience long-term breathing problems.

Mild, temporary heartbeat irregularities (arrhythmia) or rapid heartbeat (tachycardia) can occur following the conditioning regimen, particularly those that include cyclophosphamide (Cytoxan®) or carmustine (BiCNU®). Severe or long-term heart problems are rare.

Confusion

Confusion is an occasional, temporary side effect of the conditioning regimen, or of drugs used to control other side effects. Confusion can be frightening for both patients and their loved ones who observe it. It helps to remember that these problems are temporary, reversible and can usually be managed by changing the dosage or type of drug.

Muscle Spasms and Cramping

Muscle spasms are a common problem after transplant. They may be caused by an imbalance in electrolytes — minerals found in the body such as potassium, magnesium and calcium. These minerals must be maintained at certain levels to prevent organ malfunction.

Muscle spasms can often be resolved by taking magnesium, potassium, calcium or phosphate supplements. Ask your doctor to prescribe the supplement, since not all sources of these minerals are absorbed equally well by the body. If there is no electrolyte imbalance, vitamin E or a very small amount of quinine (like the amount found in tonic water) sometimes resolves or reduces the problem.

Infertility

High-dose chemotherapy and radiation cause most, but not all, patients to be infertile after transplant. Fortunately, there are options available if you wish to have children after a transplant.

Most men can bank their sperm before transplant. Sperm banking may be an option even if you had prior chemotherapy. Although you may think that you don't want children, sperm banking is worth considering in case you change your mind later on.

Discussing sperm banking with an adolescent who needs a transplant can be challenging and emotionally upsetting for the young man. Consider consulting the hospital social worker or a therapist about how best to approach this delicate matter with your child.

For women, it may be possible to collect eggs prior to transplant, fertilize them with sperm to create embryos and then freeze the embryos for later use. This procedure requires several weeks and may not be an option if you need to proceed quickly to transplant.

It is also possible to collect and freeze a woman's eggs without fertilizing them with sperm. However, unfertilized eggs are less likely to survive the freezing and thawing process than fertilized eggs.

Another experimental option for women is freezing ovarian tissue. Ovarian tissue is removed during a short, outpatient surgical procedure and then frozen. The tissue can later be implanted into a woman's ovary where it may produce eggs.

For more information about fertility preservation options before transplant go to bmtinfonet.org/preserve-fertility.

Putting Risks into Perspective

Anxiety about possible side effects is normal. It helps to put the risk of developing each side effect into perspective, and to remember that most are temporary and completely reversible. Counselors are available at most transplant centers to help you cope with anxiety. It pays to take advantage of these resources.

> "Be prepared for complications. Very few things will happen just as described. There are many possible complications. No one gets all of them, but most get some of them. Learn to separate those that are serious, but reversible, from those that are truly life-threatening."

To learn more, go to our website at:

bmtinfonet.org/conditioning-regimen

Chapter Eight

INFECTION

Six months after my transplant, I developed a herpes zoster infection, also known as shingles. I was hospitalized for ten days. That was hard. I was just getting back on my feet and wham! — I'm back in the hospital again.

Marilyn Rossen, 11-year transplant survivor

The air we breathe, the food we eat, the items we touch — everything we contact in daily life is a potential source of bacteria, viruses or fungi that can cause infection. For a normal, healthy individual these daily encounters with sources of infection are not a major problem. Our immune system protects us from infection.

For transplant patients, however, it's a different story. The high-dose chemotherapy and/or radiation administered prior to transplant not only destroys diseased cells, but temporarily disrupts the patient's immune system as well.

Skin and mucous membranes that line the mouth, nose and intestines are the body's first line of defense against infection, and may be damaged by the conditioning regimen. White blood cells, part of the body's internal defense team, are also destroyed.

Special proteins, called antibodies, that normally help destroy bacteria and viruses are depleted. Until the transplanted stem cells begin producing new white blood cells, you will be very vulnerable to infection.

Although post-transplant infections are a serious cause for concern, great strides have been made to better manage and prevent them.

Bacterial Infections

Bacteria are microscopic organisms that invade tissues and multiply rapidly. Bacteria can cause infections anywhere in the body and are the usual cause of ear and sinus infections, as well as bronchitis in the lungs.

Bacteria secrete poisonous chemicals called toxins that interfere with normal organ functions. Toxins can, among other things, cause shock or low blood pressure that can lead to death if sufficient oxygen is not provided to the heart or brain.

Bacteria can also disrupt normal organ functions by their sheer number. Some pneumonias, for example, are caused by rapidly multiplying bacteria that fill up the spaces in lungs where air is normally absorbed into the body.

> The first two-to-four weeks after a transplant are a critical time. Although the risk of infection steadily declines once the stem cells begin producing new white blood cells, your immune system will not completely recover and function normally for six months to a year, or longer, after the transplant.

Bacterial infections are most common during the first two-to-four weeks after transplant. The infections occur most often in the intestines, on the skin and in the mouth. They also occasionally occur in the bladder or lungs.

To combat bacterial infections, antibiotics are usually given during the first few weeks after transplant if the patient's temperature rises above 100.5°F. You may also receive an oral antibiotic before the first fever to try to prevent an infection. You will bathe or shower daily to remove bacteria from your skin. To avoid cuts in your mouth through which bacteria, fungi or viruses can enter your body, you'll use a soft toothbrush to clean your teeth and gums.

Hospital staff and others who come in contact with you will carefully wash their hands with antiseptic soap or alcohol gel, since hands are a primary carrier of infection. Flowers and plants (both live and dried) may not be permitted in your room while your immune system is weak. Fresh fruits and vegetables may be eliminated from your diet until your immune system is functioning normally. When detected promptly and treated with antibiotics, bacterial infections are usually well managed.

Fungal Infections

Fungi are primitive life forms that we encounter daily. Bread mold is an example of a common fungus. Most are harmless and some, such as the fungus called Candida, normally reside in our bodies.

Fungal infections are less common than bacterial infections in the first few weeks after transplant but are very difficult to treat. While the widespread use of antibiotics after transplant has reduced the incidence of harmful bacterial infections, these antibiotics can also destroy beneficial bacteria in your body that keep fungi in check.

At some transplant centers, special air-filtering equipment is installed in patient rooms to remove fungi from the air. Eliminating fresh plants, fruits and vegetables from the patient's environment may also reduce the risk of fungal infections. Patients who have continuous fevers after taking antibiotics are usually given an anti-fungal drug to help prevent fungal infections.

Candida and aspergillus are the most common fungal infections after transplant. Candida live in the intestines, mouth and vagina. A drug called fluconazole (Diflucan®) may be used to control Candida infections.

Aspergillus infections occur most often in the sinus passages or the lungs and can cause pneumonia. The aspergillus fungus is frequently found around construction sites or where buildings are being remodeled. It has also been identified in marijuana and is not killed by burning or cooking marijuana. Voriconazole (Vfend®), posaconazole (Noxafil®) and isavuconazonium sulfate (Cresemba®) have shown effectiveness in treating aspergillus infections.

A fungus called pneumocystis jirovecii (formerly called pneumocystis carinii) is found in the trachea (windpipe) of healthy humans. When a person's immune system is suppressed, this fungus can enter the lungs and grow into tiny cysts which can cause pneumonia. Trimethoprim/sulfamethoxazole (Bactrim® or Septra®), atovaquone (Mepron®), dapsone and pentamidine (Nebupent®) are used to treat pneumocystis jiroveci pneumonia.

Once blood counts return to normal levels, the risk of fungal infection drops dramatically. Overall, serious fungal infections are rare following an autologous transplant.

Viral Infections

Viruses are tiny organisms, smaller than bacteria, that are not self-sufficient. They must invade other organisms, such as human cells, to survive. Viruses tinker with the genetic machinery of the host cell, turning it into a factory to produce more of the virus. The virus eventually destroys or cripples the host cell and moves on to neighboring cells to continue the process.

Infections caused by viruses are very difficult to treat. Several antiviral agents such as acyclovir and ganciclovir are useful, but the number of viruses they effectively treat is small. Viral infections after transplant occur either as a result of exposure to a new virus or reactivation of an old virus that was already in the patient's body.

The risk of developing a serious viral infection following an autologous transplant is low. The viral infections that occur most are caused by the herpes simplex virus (HSV) or varicella zoster virus (VZV).

Herpes Simplex (HSV)

Herpes simplex infections are caused by two separate viruses: herpes I and herpes II. Although both viruses can cause an infection in any part of the body, the herpes I virus usually causes painful fever blisters in and around the mouth. The herpes II virus usually causes painful blisters on the genitalia or rectum.

An estimated 70 percent of Americans are exposed to the herpes I virus, usually during childhood. The virus is highly contagious and is usually transmitted through contact with people who have active herpes sores on their mouth. Herpes II, on the other hand, is usually transmitted through sexual intercourse with an infected partner.

Herpes infections often recur after the initial episode. The virus can lay dormant in the body for many years, flaring up from time to time.

When a herpes infection occurs, it is usually during the first month after transplant. Herpes simplex responds well to treatment with antiviral agents such as acyclovir. Most centers give patients acyclovir before a herpes infection develops which has greatly reduced the incidence of herpes infections after transplant.

Varicella Zoster Virus (VZV)

Varicella zoster virus (VZV) is often referred to as herpes zoster or shingles. It is the same virus that causes chicken pox. VZV is seen most often in patients being treated for leukemia, lymphoma or Hodgkin lymphoma.

A VZV infection can cause an itching, blistering skin rash along any one of the body's nerve branches. The nerve endings under the skin are infected and can cause great pain.

A VZV infection can also develop in the nerve to the eye, called the ophthalmic nerve, causing a painful rash on the forehead and eyelids. If not treated promptly, the infection can damage the eye.

VZV infections may be treated with oral doses of famciclovir (Famvir®) or valacyclovir (Valtrex®), or acyclovir given intravenously. They are quite contagious, and some patients must be admitted to the hospital to be treated.

The pain associated with a VZV infection can be significantly reduced if you call your doctor the day the rash first appears. Drugs such as acetaminophen (Tylenol®), codeine or morphine may help control pain. Early treatment can significantly reduce how long a VZV infection lasts.

A VZV infection can occur more than once after transplant. The itching and pain associated with a VZV infection can continue long after all clinical signs of the disease disappear. Some patients require prolonged use of medications to treat the nerve pain from a VZV infection.

Since VZV infections are highly contagious, you should avoid people with chicken pox or a VZV infection for the first year after transplant.

Recently, a VZV vaccination called Shingrix was shown to be effective in preventing zoster infections in patients undergoing autologous transplantation. This vaccine series can start as early as two months after transplant. The other available VZV vaccines should not be given until two years after transplant.

Cytomegalovirus (CMV)

Occasionally, a patient will develop a CMV infection after an autologous transplant. CMV infections can occur in different organs including the liver, colon, eyes or lungs. CMV pneumonia is particularly worrisome because it is very difficult to treat.

Approximately one-third to two-thirds of the general population are exposed to CMV during their lifetime. Doctors can test your blood prior to transplant to see if CMV is present. If it is not, care will be taken to prevent exposure to CMV before, during and after the transplant. Filtering blood products given to you to remove most of the white blood cells reduces the risk of a CMV infection.

Other Viruses

Common viruses, such as those that cause a cold (rhinovirus, coronovirus, parainfluenza virus) or the flu (influenza virus) can cause serious infections for patients up to a year after transplant. Other viruses such as adenovirus, papovavirus, Epstein-Barr virus (EBV), respiratory syncytial virus (RSV) and human papilloma virus (HPV) can also create problems after transplant, although the incidence of these infections is quite low.

Adenovirus and RSV infections can cause pneumonia. Adenovirus can cause an infection in the kidneys or gastrointestinal tract. Ribavirin (Virazole®) is effective in treating both of these viruses.

The likelihood of developing these viral infections can be reduced by limiting contact with the public after transplant, particularly people with the flu or a cold, and by meticulous hand washing. Some centers require a brief period of isolation from the general public after transplant to reduce the risk of becoming infected with these viruses.

Protozoan Infections

Protozoa are single-cell parasites that feed on organisms such as human cells to survive. Although infections from protozoa are less common than bacterial or viral infections, they can pose serious problems for transplant patients.

An infection called toxoplasmosis occasionally develops in patients after transplant. Toxoplasmosis is caused by a protozoan called toxoplasma gondii which is often transmitted by cat feces. Toxoplasmosis may infect the brain, eyes, muscles, liver and/or lungs. A painful, inflamed retina in the eye is a common manifestation of the disease which, without prompt treatment, can result in damage to the eye. With early diagnosis and proper treatment, toxoplasmosis is treatable.

Preventing Infection

Although it may be tempting to throw caution to the wind after a transplant, it's best not to take chances. Bacteria, viruses, fungi and protozoa that are harmless to most people can cause a serious infection in someone whose immune system has not yet fully recovered.

Your medical team will give you guidelines to help prevent infections. The most important of these is frequent hand washing with antibacterial soap or an alcohol-based hand sanitizer before eating and preparing food.

You should also wash your hands after:

- changing diapers (if you are permitted to do so)
- touching plants or dirt (if you are permitted to do so)
- going to the bathroom
- touching animals
- touching bodily fluids or items that might have come in contact with bodily fluids such as clothing, bedding or toilets
- going outdoors or to a public place
- removing gloves
- collecting or depositing garbage (if you are permitted to do so)

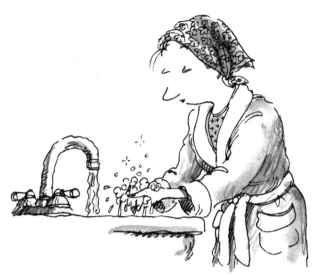

- before and after touching catheters and wounds

During the first six months after transplant, many transplant centers recommend that you avoid:

- crowds or people who have infections

- people who have recently been vaccinated with live virus vaccines such as chicken pox

- changing a baby's diapers

- gardening

- walking, wading, swimming or playing in ponds or lakes

- construction sites and remodeling projects while you are at risk for infections

- well water that has not been treated

If You Have Pets

Rules vary among transplant centers as to whether or not you can have pets in the home while you are recovering. Consult your transplant center for its guidelines. You may be advised to:

- avoid contact with an animal that is ill

- not adopt ill or juvenile pets (juvenile pets are more likely to scratch than mature pets)

- avoid reptiles such as lizards, snakes, turtles and iguanas and items they touch

- avoid chicks and ducklings

- not handle exotic pets such as monkeys or chinchillas

- not clean litter boxes or cages or dispose of animal waste

- not clean fish tanks

Your transplant center may also recommend that you:

- feed pets only high quality commercial food or thoroughly cooked human food

- do not touch bird droppings

- do not place cat litter boxes in areas of the house where food is prepared or eaten

- keep cats indoors and not adopt stray cats

- cover backyard sandboxes to prevent cats from using them as a litter box

At the first sign of fever or infection, call your physician. Infections are most easily treated when caught early. Infections you formerly ignored can be serious problems after transplant. Taking precautions to guard against infection can be a nuisance, but it can also save your life.

Re-vaccination

After an autologous transplant, antibodies that previously protected you against disease may be depleted. Guidelines from the Centers for Disease Control (CDC) suggest that patients be re-vaccinated for diphtheria, tetanus, pneumococcus, hemophilus, influenza type B and polio infections beginning six-to-eighteen months after transplant. The CDC recommends waiting until two years after transplant to receive the MMR vaccine for measles, mumps and rubella.

Your transcript team may recommend that you get the flu vaccine starting at six months after transplant. You should discuss with your transplant doctor the appropriate timing for you to get re-vaccinated.

For more information go to our website at:

bmtinfonet.org/prevent-infection

Chapter Nine

NUTRITION

After my transplant, I was the nausea queen. You name it, I could throw it up. For a while, all I could handle was Carnation Instant Breakfast®. Then I worked my way up to Cap'n Crunch®— box after box of it — then coffee and beer, and finally, at long last, a normal diet.

Judith Miller, 6-year transplant survivor

We all need food and water to thrive. The calories in food provide the fuel our organs and tissues need to grow and function. Protein-rich foods enable the body to build and repair muscle and body tissue. Vitamins and minerals keep blood, skin and the nervous system functioning properly.

Transplant patients have unique nutritional requirements. Prior to transplant, patients undergo high-dose chemotherapy and/or total body irradiation (TBI) to destroy their disease. This severely stresses the body's organs and tissues. In order to repair any organ or tissue damage that might occur and to fight fever, patients need to increase their intake of calories and protein.

Typically, transplant patients require 50-60 percent more calories and twice as much protein in their diets than healthy individuals of similar age and gender. The need for more calories and protein persists at least one-to-two months after transplant.

Changing Diet Before Transplant

Some patients consider making major dietary changes before their transplant. Some attempt to shed excess weight. Others eat foods that have been associated with a lower incidence of cancer. Still others turn to macrobiotic or other diets that restrict the types of foods consumed.

If you are considering changing your diet, ask your doctor for a referral to a registered dietitian who can evaluate the nutritional adequacy of the new diet. Some diets, such as macrobiotic diets, contain lower amounts of protein and other nutrients than are needed by a recovering transplant patient.

Using certain herbs, roots or over the counter dietary supplements can be dangerous for people undergoing transplantation. Consult your doctor or dietitian before using these products.

Quick weight loss is also usually discouraged. Since patients often lose weight while undergoing treatment, limiting food intake before a transplant could cause a serious nutrient deficiency.

Nutrition after Transplant

For the first three months after transplant, patients are usually advised to avoid foods that may contain organisms that might cause infection. Most transplant centers have specific recommendations on foods to avoid which may include:

- raw or undercooked meat
- dishes that may contain undercooked meat, such as casseroles
- raw or undercooked eggs or foods that might contain them
- raw or undercooked seafood, such as sushi
- unroasted raw nuts or unshelled nuts
- meats and cheeses from a deli
- miso and tempeh products
- milk products that are not pasteurized including Mexican-style soft cheeses such as queso fresco and queso blanco

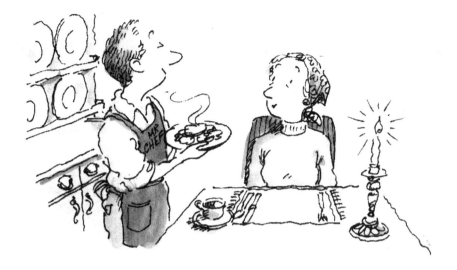

- cheeses with mold such as blue cheese, Brie, Camembert, Gorgonzola, Roquefort and Stilton

- soft cheeses such as feta, goat's cheese, and farmer's cheese

- smoked, uncooked refrigerated fish such as nova lox

- pickled seafood

- raw honey

- salad bars and buffets

Some transplant centers include fresh fruits and vegetables on the list of foods to avoid, while others permit them provided they are thoroughly washed. Consult your transplant team to learn which dietary restrictions apply to you and for how long.

Consuming sufficient calories, protein and fluids can be difficult particularly during the first few weeks after transplant. Mouth sores, nausea, vomiting, dry mouth, diarrhea, constipation, depression and fatigue can make mealtimes unappealing. Certain medications can also cause a loss of appetite.

Some patients must be fed intravenously during this period to ensure they receive sufficient calories, protein, vitamins, minerals and fluids. The intravenous feeding is called total parenteral nutrition (TPN) or hyperalimentation and may supply all your nutritional requirements or supplement those you are able to consume on your own.

Often, eating problems can be overcome without resorting to the use of TPN. The following sections describe common eating problems after transplant and tips for managing them.

Mouth and Throat Sores

Mouth and throat sores are common after transplant. They may be caused by chemotherapy, total body irradiation or infection. If mouth sores are a problem for you try:

- lukewarm or cold foods, rather than hot foods

- cooking foods until tender and soft

- drinking through a straw to bypass mouth sores

- high-protein, high-calorie foods to speed healing of the sores

- a liquid or blenderized diet, or a complete nutrition supplement such as Ensure®, Boost® or Carnation Instant Breakfast®

- soft foods such as creamed soups, pasteurized cheese, mashed potatoes, cooked eggs, custards, puddings, gelatin, soft canned fruit, cooked cereals and pasteurized eggnog

- cold foods such as milk shakes, ice cream, cottage cheese, yogurt, slushes and watermelon

- soft, frozen foods such as popsicles, ice cream and frozen yogurt

- pasteurized nectars and fruit flavored beverages instead of acidic juices

If you develop mouth or throat sores, avoid:

- tart or acidic foods and beverages such as citrus fruits and juices, pineapple juice and tomato products

- salty food, including broth

- strong spices such as peppers, chili powder, nutmeg and cloves

- coarse foods such as raw fruits and vegetables, dry toast, grainy cereals and breads and crunchy snacks

- alcoholic beverages and mouthwashes that contain alcohol

- extremely hot foods or beverages

If the mouth pain is severe, ask your transplant team for pain medication.

Dry Mouth

Dry mouth is a common side effect of total body irradiation, anti-nausea medications and antihistamines. If a dry mouth is making eating difficult, try the following:

- Add sauces, gravies, broth and dressings to foods.

- Suck ice chips, popsicles, sugarless gum or hard candies to keep your mouth moist.

- Add citric acid to your diet to stimulate saliva production, unless you have mouth or throat sores. Citric acid is in oranges, orange juice, lemons, lemonade and sugarless lemon drops. You can also add lemon to tea, water and soda.

- Drink clear liquids with your meals.

- Ask your dietitian or doctor about commercial saliva substitutes such as Salivart®, Mouth Kote® and Biotène®.

Avoid eating:

- meats without sauces

- bread products, crackers and dry cakes

- very hot foods and beverages

- alcoholic beverages and mouthwashes that contain alcohol

Changes in Taste

Total body irradiation, chemotherapy and some pain medications can make foods you normally enjoy taste unpleasant. To overcome this problem, try eating or drinking:

- cold food and beverages

- strongly flavored foods such as chocolate, lasagna, spaghetti or barbecued foods, unless you also have mouth or throat sores

- tart or spicy foods, unless you also have mouth or throat sores

- fluids with your meal to rinse away any bad taste

- protein foods without strong odors, such as poultry, eggs and dairy products rather than those with strong odors such as beef and fish

- sauces with foods

- meats with something sweet, such as cranberry sauce, jelly or applesauce

- new seasonings or adding sugar or salt to enhance the taste

If food has a metallic taste, try using plastic eating utensils.

Thick Saliva

Total body irradiation and dehydration can cause thick saliva. If thick saliva is interfering with your eating, try the following:

- Drink club soda (seltzer) or hot tea with lemon.

- Suck sugarless sour lemon drops.

- Eat a lighter breakfast if you have mucous build up in the morning, and bigger meals in the afternoon and evening.

- Rinse frequently with a saline solution (one quart water with 1/2 teaspoon salt and one-to-two teaspoons baking soda).

- Drink lots of fluids.

- Eat soft, tender foods such as cooked fish and chicken, eggs, noodles, thinned cereals and blenderized fruits and vegetables diluted to a very thin consistency.

- Eat small, frequent meals.

- Drink diluted juices, broth-based soups and fruit-flavored beverages.

- Switch to a liquid diet if the problem is severe.

Avoid eating:

- meats that require chewing
- bread products
- oily foods
- thick cream soups
- thick hot cereals
- nectars

Nausea and Vomiting

High-dose chemotherapy, total body irradiation, infection, some medications and mucous drainage from your mouth and sinuses can trigger nausea and vomiting.

If nausea is interfering with your ability to eat, try eating:

- small, frequent meals
- dry crackers or toast, especially before movement, such as getting out of bed, unless you have mouth sores
- cold foods, rather than warm foods, because they tend to have less odor
- low-fat foods such as cooked vegetables, canned fruit, baked skinless chicken, sherbet, fruit ice, popsicles, gelatin, pretzels, vanilla wafers and angel food cake
- clear, cool liquids such as carbonated beverages, flavored gelatin, popsicles and ice cubes made of a favorite liquid
- liquids sipped slowly through a straw
- small amounts of liquid frequently throughout the day

If you are hospitalized, you can:

- request antinausea medication 30 minutes before your meal
- ask that food trays be brought to you without covers on the plates so you're not overwhelmed by the smell when the cover is removed

Avoid eating or drinking:

- spicy foods

- foods that are overly sweet

- strong smelling foods

- foods that are high in fat

- hot liquids with meals

- liquids on an empty stomach

If you are nauseated, avoid lying flat on your back after eating. This can make the problem worse. If you need rest, sit or recline with your head elevated. Avoid perfumes and other strong-smelling cosmetics.

Ask for medication to control the nausea if it is severe.

Lack of Appetite/Weight Loss

Many transplant patients experience weight loss and lack of appetite for a period of time. Possible causes include total body irradiation, chemotherapy, infection, depression and fatigue. If you don't have an appetite for food try eating or drinking:

- small, frequent, high-calorie meals

- high-nutrient liquids such as juice or milk instead of low-calorie drinks like coffee, tea or diet soda

- nutrient-dense, high-calorie foods like:
  - pasteurized cheese, whole milk and ice cream
  - eggs
  - avocados
  - olives
  - Greek yogurt
  - hummus
  - trail mix
  - fruit smoothies
  - protein powder
  - dried fruit
  - peanut butter

- wheat germ
- nuts
- fruits

- protein supplements such as Promod® or complete nutrition supplements such as Ensure®, Boost®, Carnation Instant Breakfast® or Sustacal®, provided they have been approved by your dietitian

- non-fat dry milk added to casseroles or cooked cereals

You can also try:

- creating a pleasant mealtime atmosphere with colorful place settings, varied food colors and textures and soft music

- engaging in light exercise to stimulate your appetite

- addressing any psychological problems that may be causing the loss of appetite

- asking your doctor about medications that may improve your appetite

Diarrhea

Diarrhea can occur following total body irradiation or high-dose chemotherapy. It may also be caused by an infection called *Clostridium difficile* colitis or C. Diff, for short. Some antibiotics and oral medications, such as magnesium salts or metoclopramide (Reglan®) can also cause diarrhea. In other cases, diarrhea may be caused by infection or lactose intolerance — an inability to digest the lactose in milk products.

If you are experiencing diarrhea try eating or drinking:

- smaller amounts of food at each meal

- extra fluids to prevent dehydration

- fluids between meals rather than with meals

- foods and beverages that are high in potassium such as:
  - ripe bananas
  - potatoes without the skin
  - tomato juice, Gatorade®, Pedialyte®, Powerade®, orange juice and pasteurized peach and pear nectar

- o baked fish, chicken and ground beef
- o well cooked eggs
- o well-cooked vegetables (but not beans, broccoli, cauliflower or cabbage)
- o canned fruit
- o white rice
- o white bread

Avoid eating:

- bran or whole grain cereals and breads

- raw vegetables

- fruits with skin and seeds

- popcorn, seeds and nuts

- carbonated beverages

- beans, broccoli, cauliflower and cabbage

- chewing gum

- spicy foods

- foods with rich gravies or sauces

- foods and drinks with caffeine such as coffee, tea, chocolate, colas and other caffeinated soft drinks

- dairy products unless they are treated with Lactaid®

Do not take over-the-counter medications like Imodium® unless approved by your doctor, since these drugs sometimes make a colon infection worse.

Constipation

Some chemotherapy drugs, opioid pain medications and antinausea medications cause constipation. Try eating or drinking:

- warm beverages

- high-fiber foods such as well washed raw fruits and vegetables, whole wheat bread and cereals and dried fruit. Be sure you drink plenty of fluids while eating these foods.

- warm prune juice or stewed prunes

Light exercise may also help with constipation. Ask your doctor about stool softeners or laxatives if the problem persists for more than two days.

Herbs, Botanicals and Supplements

Until your immune system has fully recovered, you should avoid taking any herb, botanical or supplement without your doctor's approval. Some of these products can:

- reduce the effectiveness of other drugs you are taking

- cause a serious infection due to inadequate purification of the product or extra ingredients it contains

- damage your liver, kidneys or other organs

- make gastrointestinal problems worse

- interfere with blood clotting

Herbal and botanical products to avoid while your immune system is recovering include:

- alfalfa

- borage

- chaparral

- Chinese herbs

- coltsfoot

- comfrey

- DHEA

- dieter's tea (including senna, aloe, rhubarb root, buckthorn, cascara, castor oil)

- ephedra or mahuang

- groundsel or life root

- heliotrope or valerian

- kava kava

- laetrile (apricot pits)

- licorice root

- lobelia

- L-tryptophan

- maté tea

- pau d'arco

- pennyroyal

- sassafras

- St. John's wort

- yohimbe and yohimbine

If your platelet count is low, you should avoid garlic pill supplements (cooking with regular garlic is fine) and gingko biloba, which can interfere with blood clotting.

Check with your doctor to see whether there are other herbs, supplements or botanicals that you should also avoid while your immune system is recovering, or while you are on medications that may interact with them.

To learn more, go to our website at:

bmtinfonet.org/nutrition

Chapter Ten

RELIEVING PAIN

I was given a wonderful little button that allowed me to self-dispense morphine every five minutes. I pushed it a lot. I don't remember much more about that week — I've blocked it out. It's a fog and I'm glad.

Jim King, 28-year transplant survivor

For some people about to undergo a transplant, fear of pain is greater than worries about potential complications. In this chapter, we'll examine the type of pain patients sometimes experience and various drugs used to control it. We'll also discuss some non-drug techniques that can help provide relief.

What is Pain?

Today's pain specialists agree that pain is whatever a patient says it is, whenever, wherever and to whatever degree he or she says it occurs. The sensation of pain is influenced by physical factors, such as tissue damage, as well as psychological, social and environmental factors.

Two different people with the same amount of tissue damage may experience very different levels of pain. Moreover, each person's body absorbs and processes pain medications differently. Thus, the amount of medication required to ease one person's pain may differ greatly from that required to ease another's pain. In short, pain is a very personal experience requiring a highly individualized response from the medical team.

Pain can be described as acute or chronic. Acute pain, usually due to tissue damage, lasts days to weeks and ends once the tissue damage is healed. Most pain experienced by transplant patients is acute pain. The word acute does not mean that the pain is sharper or more uncomfortable. It simply refers to the length of time over which pain occurs.

Chronic pain persists over months or years and is caused by irreparable tissue damage, nerve damage or by unknown causes. Often, chronic pain can only be controlled; its source cannot be eliminated.

How Pain is Experienced

The pain experienced by patients undergoing an autologous transplant is usually caused by temporary inflammation of tissues or nerves. Sensors at the tissue or nerve site detect the physical damage and transmit distress signals to the brain.

Suffering is the person's response to those pain signals. The degree of suffering varies greatly according to the person's emotional and physical condition at the time pain is experienced. Fatigue, depression, anxiety, physical weakness, memories of how well the pain was managed in the past and fears about the cause of the pain can increase the suffering associated with pain.

Blocking Pain Signals

The sensation of pain is relieved by blocking the pain signals with drugs, or with a combination of drug and non-drug therapies.

The most commonly used pain medications for transplant patients are opioids. Opioids include drugs such as morphine and hydromorphone (Dilaudid®). Non-opioid drugs such as aspirin, ibuprofen and acetaminophen are often not strong enough to provide sufficient pain relief for transplant patients.

At some transplant centers, massage, application of heat or cold to the affected area, exercise, relaxation, visualization, hypnosis and distraction are used to enhance the relief provided by pain medications.

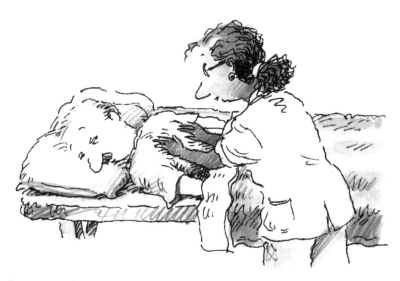

Pain Experienced by Transplant Patients

Each person's transplant experience is unique. Some people experience only mild discomfort and need only small amounts of pain medication. Others experience more significant pain and require more medication to control it.

Mouth and Skin Sores

Painful mouth sores are common in transplant patients. Medications such as Lidocaine® can be used like a mouth wash to control the discomfort. In many cases, an opioid such as morphine is given to provide additional relief.

High-dose chemotherapy and radiation can sometimes cause skin sores. Opioids are typically used to control the pain. If a burning sensation accompanies the pain, aloe vera gel (not with an alcohol base), Eucerin® or Silvaderm™/Lidocaine® cream may be applied directly to the skin.

Medical Procedures

Certain medical procedures can cause temporary discomfort. A bone marrow biopsy is an example. In this procedure, a needle is inserted into the rear of the hip bone to withdraw a tiny sample of bone marrow. While the area around the bone can be numbed, it's not possible to numb the bone itself. An uncomfortable scraping sensation and pressure are common with bone marrow biopsies.

Anxiety about the procedure can be reduced by pre-medicating you with a small amount of Versed® or Ativan® to relax you, and a small dosage of opioid to help relieve the pain. Don't be embarrassed to ask for pre-medication to ease your anxiety if you're fearful about a bone marrow biopsy.

In some cases, it may be possible for your healthcare team to briefly sedate you with powerful, short-term general anesthetics, in addition to local anesthetics, so that you are not fully conscious while the procedure is taking place. This technique, called conscious sedation, requires an anesthesiologist and more elaborate preparation, such as withholding food and drink for six-to-seven hours prior to the procedure. If you are anxious about painful medical procedures, inquire about this technique.

Growth Factors

Growth factors used to speed the recovery of white blood cells after transplant can cause mild to moderate bone pain, muscle pain and headaches. In most cases, the pain can be controlled with acetaminophen (Tylenol®) or an antihistamine such as Claritin® and usually ends when you stop taking these drugs. If the pain is severe, opioids may be used to relieve it.

Peripheral Neuropathy

Peripheral neuropathy is a symptom of nerve damage that sometimes occurs after transplant. Some patients, such as those with multiple myeloma, may already have peripheral neuropathy before going to transplant.

Peripheral neuropathy can cause pain or tingling in the hands and feet. The discomfort may be greater at night or in cold weather.

If you are experiencing symptoms of peripheral neuropathy, consult a neurologist. Although it is not possible to cure the nerve damage, drugs such as pregabalin (Lyrica®), gabapentin and duloxetine (Cymbalta®) are available to treat the pain. Non-drug therapies such as transcutaneous electrical nerve stimulation (TENS), biofeedback and hypnosis may also help.

If you have peripheral neuropathy, it is important to check your feet daily for signs of ulcers and infections. If peripheral neuropathy is affecting your balance, physical therapy may help.

You can learn more about managing peripheral neuropathy online at bmtinfonet.org/neuropathy.

Identifying the Cause of Pain

In order to properly treat pain, its cause must be identified. Most pain has a physical cause that can either be seen by a physician or deduced based on the patient's history and description of the pain.

Sometimes a physical cause for the pain is not readily apparent. This does not mean that the pain is any less real or less urgent to relieve. Pain experts agree that when you say that you are experiencing pain, it's important for your healthcare team to take that complaint seriously and attempt to relieve it, whether or not a physical cause is apparent.

Notify your physician or nurse about pain as soon as it begins. It is easier to relieve pain in the early stages than after it has become severe.

There is no need to endure pain. Don't be embarrassed about asking for relief.

In fact, refusing pain medication may be harmful. Patients who are gripped by pain are often less able to do important things that are necessary for recovery, such as eating or exercising.

You can help your physician properly identify the cause of pain by being very specific about the description, intensity, location and frequency of the pain.

- Rate the pain on a scale of 0-10 (0=no pain, 10=worst pain). Is it mild, moderate or severe?

- Is it sharp or a dull ache? Does it throb? Is there a burning or itching sensation associated with it?

- Is it constant or does it only occur sometimes? How often does it occur? How long does it last?

- Is it better or worse at certain times of the day or night?

- When did it begin?

- Do certain actions such as lying down or taking a deep breath make the pain better or worse?

• How is it affecting your daily life?

The more information your doctor has about the pain, the more likely he or she will be able to identify and treat both the cause and symptoms properly.

Choosing a Drug and Dosage

The drug chosen to relieve pain will depend on the physical cause of the pain. Opioids are effective in controlling pain caused by tissue damage, such as mouth sores or a skin rash. Antidepressants and anti-convulsants may help control pain caused by nerve damage.

Some drugs are very slow acting but produce long-term pain relief. Others quickly reduce pain but are effective only for a short period of time. A combination of drugs is sometimes used to provide the best relief.

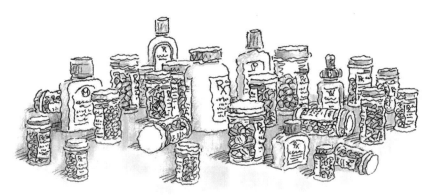

Maintaining Relief

If pain increases, the amount of pain medication may need to be increased. Some drugs, such as opioids, provide additional pain relief whenever the dosage is increased while others do not.

Increasing the amount of drugs may increase the risk of side effects. These side effects are usually minor and reversible, but you should not increase the dosage or frequency of pain medications without checking with your doctor.

While in the hospital or clinic, you may be given a Patient Controlled Analgesia (PCA) machine which allows you to administer your own pain medication, up to a safe limit, as needed. Pain relief may also be administered by a pain patch applied to the skin which delivers narcotics continuously for three days.

Fear of Addiction

One of the biggest barriers to providing patients with adequate pain relief is the fear of addiction. Thus, some opt to put up with pain rather than ask for pain medication.

Pain medication will be given to you only as long as you need it. Your care team will taper down the dosage once your pain is under control. In most cases, unless you have a history of addiction, it is unlikely that you will become addicted to pain medications.

What If Pain Continues?

Since pain relief must be tailored to each individual's needs, it may take some time before the appropriate type and level of medication can be determined. You can help your doctor by providing feedback on how well the pain medication is working.

- Has the medication provided any relief at all?

- Does the drug wear off before you're scheduled to take the next dose?

- Are you experiencing any side effects such as drowsiness, nervousness, nausea, itching or constipation?

If you feel you are not receiving adequate pain relief, don't hesitate to tell your doctor or nurse.

Non-Drug Pain Control Techniques

Olympic athletes do it. Football stars do it. In fact, everyone, at some time or another, has relied on methods to relieve discomfort that don't involve drugs.

Women preparing for childbirth often use breathing exercises to relieve pain during labor and delivery. Heat, cold, immobilization and physical therapy are commonly used by athletes to relieve pain caused by sports injuries.

While drugs are the primary source of pain relief for transplant patients, positive coping statements, distraction, relaxation, imagery, hypnosis, application of heat or cold to the affected area, massage and exercise can enhance relief.

Positive Coping Statements

Fear and a feeling of helplessness are common among transplant patients. Not only has a powerful disease taken control of their body, but they are forced to rely on a team of complete strangers to save their life. Anger and frustration over this lack of control can lead to anxiety and depression, which in turn can make it more difficult to tolerate pain.

Although these negative thoughts and feelings are normal, you may be able to exercise some control over them with positive coping statements. Focus on the various things you can do rather than those that you can't do. Take encouragement from even small accomplishments, or find something positive in each experience.

For example, if you're discouraged because the days of treatment seem to be passing slowly, try focusing on the fact that you have already successfully made it through several days, and that you are moving closer to the day of full recovery. If you experience some backsliding, e.g. your blood counts go down or your body is not responding to certain medications, remind yourself that temporary setbacks are normal and not a cause for alarm. Think about the progress you have made overall since starting your treatment and try not to measure each day against the successes of a prior day.

Some patients find that repeating encouraging phrases like prayers, or the words 'I am coping well', help.

> "I had a friend — an older gentleman — who came to my house before the transplant. He was 6'-4", had a tall crop of white hair, wore cowboy boots, lean jeans and a rope tie. He said he was going to help me relax and keep the pain from my mind. He taught me several relaxation techniques. I was always able to call him, and he'd give me some key words or phrases that helped me start relaxing until the medications arrived or until I stopped panicking."

If it is difficult to find something positive in each day's experience, ask the hospital social worker, pastoral counselor, psychologist or psychiatry staff for help. Often, they can suggest ways to cope with your frustrations and refocus your attention on more positive thoughts.

Distraction

Distraction is probably the most familiar non-drug pain control technique. Watching a movie, listening to soothing music or talking with visitors can divert your attention from discomfort and focus it on a more pleasurable experience.

Before your transplant, think about the kinds of activities that will help pass the time and provide a distraction from worry and pain. Set aside recordings of music or stories, movies with uncomplicated plots, books (simple stories or picture books may be all you can handle) or family games that you enjoy. Keep in mind that you may be groggy and your attention span may be shorter while you're taking medication.

Storytelling is an excellent distraction for children. Letting the child tell the story with you works best, but listening to stories can be helpful as well. Art projects also work well with children.

Relaxation and Imagery

Relaxation and imagery are commonly used to relieve anxiety and pain. Relaxation involves a series of muscle tensing and relaxing exercises or focused breathing exercises designed to induce a sense of calm.

Relaxation is most effective when combined with imagery. Imagery involves thinking of a pleasant, safe, relaxing place or activity that brings you happiness. Exploring this place or activity in your mind in great detail can help induce a sense of calm.

> "When I began to panic or experience discomfort, I'd close my eyes and concentrate on my own breathing until all I could hear was my breathing and heartbeat. Then I'd picture my toes and try to put them to sleep, and work my way up my legs, thighs, hips, arms and hands until I felt very heavy. Once I achieved that heaviness,

I'd try to picture a place I'd like to be and concentrate on the details. I pictured myself as sixteen-years-old, wearing a white gauzy dress, sitting with my dog on my favorite patchwork quilt in a forest glen, with the rays of the sun coming through the trees. My long hair would be blowing in the breeze, and it felt good. After that, I would be calm."

Relaxation and imagery techniques are easy to learn, but they take an initial investment of time, concentration and practice to master. They're most effective if learned in advance of your transplant when you're better able to concentrate.

Depending on the complexity of the relaxation technique and whether you're learning it alone or with guidance, it may require a few weeks of practice before you can use it effectively. Experiment with several methods until you find one that's right for you and then stick with it.

Hypnosis

Hypnosis is often used by therapists to help patients change the way they experience pain. Hypnosis may shift your focus away from the pain or shorten your perception of how long the pain lasts.

Some people have an easier time using hypnosis than others. Children appear to be more hypnotizable than adults since they are more willing to engage in fantasy. To locate a therapist in your area who is skilled in hypnosis, contact the department of behavioral medicine at a cancer center near you.

Physical Stimulation

Suffering is triggered by pain signals transmitted through the nervous system and spinal cord to the brain. One way to dull these pain signals is to provide a different, competing physical sensation.

Applying heat or cold to painful areas, for example, often masks pain signals and reduces suffering. Ice packs, however, should not be used for six months on skin that has been irradiated. Massage can also provide a soothing sensation that competes with pain signals.

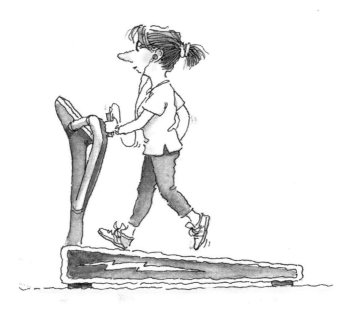

Some patients find exercise a potent pain reliever.

> "I developed a case of shingles after my transplant. I continued to have discomfort long after the sores had healed. I tried everything to control the pain including acupuncture and pain pills. Nothing worked. Finally, I began to work out at the gym seven days a week. That turned out to be the best pain relief of all."

Finding a Local Pain Specialist

After your transplant, don't hesitate to seek the help of a pain specialist if you feel your local physician is not taking your complaints of pain seriously or is unable to prescribe adequate pain medication. Most physicians have not received specialized training in pain control and some are more experienced than others in this rapidly evolving area of medicine.

Many universities and large hospitals now have special pain control programs with experts in both drug and non-drug pain control techniques who may be able to help you.

Watch a helpful video about managing pain at:

bmtinfonet.org/video-manage-pain

Chapter Eleven
FAMILY CAREGIVER

Pamper not only the patient, but the caregiver as well. Caregivers need mail, home-cooked meals, a gift certificate to their favorite store, bath gel, something they would never get themselves like music, a book, colorful socks, a gourmet candy bar — something to brighten their day and make them feel special. Even if you just send a $10 check with a note that says, 'Thought you could use a little extra something' — these things make a big difference. Long after the transplant, memories of the experience will linger with the caregiver. Out of the blue, write or call. It's important that caregivers know you're still thinking of them.

Sarah Routman, mother of a 22-month-old transplant patient

An autologous transplant is a difficult experience for patients and family members alike. As everyone's attention focuses on saving the patient's life, the needs of one of the patient's most important partners — the family member or friend who is the primary caregiver — are often underestimated.

An autologous transplant is not a procedure you can navigate alone. Most transplant teams require you to have a full-time caregiver to help during transplant and the recovery period, and will not allow you to go forward with a transplant unless a caregiver has been identified.

Typically, a close family member serves as the caregiver. If you do not have a close family member or friend who can serve as your caregiver, you may need to reach out to extended family members or friends for help, or hire a temporary caregiver. Some patients assemble a team of caregivers.

Caring for a transplant patient is physically challenging and emotionally draining. Watching as a loved one undergoes difficult medical procedures taxes even the most optimistic and healthy caregiver. Helping other family members cope adds to the burden.

Why a Full-Time Family Caregiver?

While you are undergoing treatment, you will be too ill and weak to manage medical and household affairs without help for several weeks. A full-time family caregiver can help ensure that you get prompt medical attention and that your home is a safe environment.

While you are in the hospital, your family caregiver will need to:

- alert the medical team about any changes in your condition

- provide you with emotional support

- advocate for your needs and help with decision-making

- communicate with family and friends

After you are discharged from the hospital, you caregiver will also need to:

- transport you to the outpatient clinic daily or weekly

- keep track of medical appointments

- make sure you take your many medications according to schedule

- take care of dressings and the central venous catheter

- report changes in your condition to the medical team

- monitor you for signs of infection and other complications

- encourage you to eat

- in some cases, provide you with intravenous medications

- clean and cook according to the guidelines provided by the transplant team

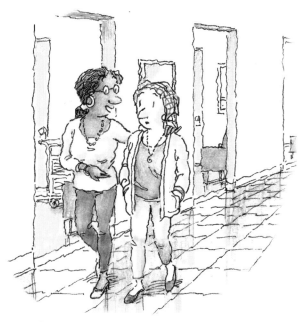

- protect you from sources of infection, such as visitors with colds or those who have been around sick people

- help you move around safely

Taking Time to Recharge

In order to provide the best possible care for the patient, caregivers need to take time off for themselves to recharge. There are many things you can do to relieve the stress of caregiving, get a clear head and find a little bit of perspective. Whether you choose to go for a walk, take in a movie, visit with friends or just nap, taking time for yourself is essential, say former caregivers.

> "Even though you may not want to or think you need to, getting away from the caregiving world for even half an hour is important. One person, even a workaholic, can't handle this situation alone."

> "You're going to feel tired, frustrated, even annoyed at your loved one sometimes, and that's OK. It's a very stressful time for everyone and you are only human. Even though you love the person going through the transplant, there will be days when you are just plain tired of

the hospital, the disease and the treatment. Try to take some time for yourself. Go for a walk outside. Get away from the hospital if just for a few minutes. Write in a journal, read a book, work on a project. (I put photos in an album.) You are not being selfish. You have to take time for yourself, in order to really help your loved one."

You need to take time for yourself even when the transplant is over and the patient returns home. At home, you will have to assume many tasks that were handled by nurses in the hospital or clinic. It is critical to pace yourself because you may be giving care intensively for a long time.

"When my wife came home from the hospital, caring for her was even harder than it was while she was hospitalized. I no longer had nurses and doctors on hand to monitor her, and I had to be constantly vigilant to detect problems. That was a lot of stress. During times when the patient is not in danger, try to take a few days away for yourself. You will be under a lot of stress for the long haul, and you need to get some relief."

Some caregivers find that classes on caring for a chronically ill patient, offered at some hospitals or health agencies, helps.

"The transplant center instructed me on things specific to transplant patients, like how to take care of the catheter. But courses for caregivers of chronically ill patients at our local hospital were also helpful. They taught the basics of caring for chronically ill patients — like how to help them without disrupting the household, how to help them walk without injuring yourself, etc. It was basic information that would be covered in a nursing assistance course."

Taking Care of Physical Well-Being

A caregiver is only effective if he or she is in good physical condition. Constantly overdoing it can backfire. Eat well balanced meals, exercise and sleep when you can. You need to stay well in order to take proper care of the patient.

"Learn, develop and practice good self-care skills prior to the transplant. Once the transplant begins, your primary attention will be on the patient, and you'll have little time or energy left to learn these skills."

"I knew from the start I was in for a long haul and had to take care of myself. I set 11 p.m. as my curfew and let my wife know I had to leave the hospital then so I could sleep and come back in the morning refreshed. I pretty much stuck to that except for those nights when things weren't going well. When I stayed overnight at the hospital, I really paid for it for the next two-to-three days."

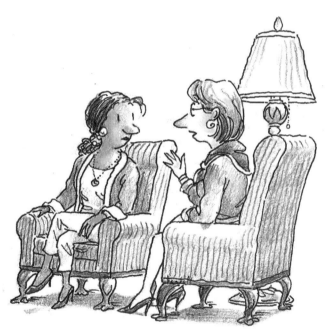

Managing Feelings

One of the complexities of being a caregiver is that it's not neutral: caregivers are taking care of patients about whom they care deeply. People who have done it stress the importance of having a forum for talking about your feelings and fears apart from the patient. Don't count on the patient to understand your emotional needs. Lean on others for support.

"Don't get so caught up worrying about everyone else that you don't deal with your own feelings and fears. Find a counselor or someone who understands what you are going through and talk your feelings out. Allow yourself to cry. I didn't do this, and after several months of anxiety, I started having physical symptoms. If you don't deal with your feelings, they will deal with you."

Find someone who is a good listener, who will let you talk about your feelings. Some caregivers find that a special friend or small circle of friends works well. Others find the families of other transplant patients most helpful. Professional counseling or talks with clergy help many caregivers deal with the experience.

"It helps to have your own network of friends whose number one concern is how you are doing. The caregiver is so busy worrying about what the patient needs, she often doesn't recognize her own feelings. I had a few family members and friends who would contact me periodically to see how I was doing. I kept a diary and would send it to them, and they'd call or write in response. Their calls made me sit down and think about how I was really feeling."

"I frequently talked with other families on the transplant unit. They were in as much pain as I was and understood what I was going through. We all helped each other. We were one big family."

"Seek counseling and the help of a spiritual advisor before the transplant begins. This experience changed my belief system on a very deep level and in ways I could not have predicted. I was grateful to have an already established channel for expressing and discussing these changes."

BMT InfoNet can link you with others who have been through the caregiving experience. Phone 888-597-7674 or go to bmtinfonet.org/caring-connection.

Accepting Help

Planning for the long haul includes inviting and accepting help from others. Many people assume that the transplant is simply their own problem to manage. Yet taking care of a very sick patient and managing the usual household and work chores is more than most people can handle.

Extended family members and friends often truly want to help, but don't know what would be most appreciated. Figure out what people are good at and give them jobs that suit their temperament and skills. If someone enjoys physical activity, let that friend cut the grass. Good cooks can prepare meals. Parents of your children's friends can help shuttle them to school and after school activities. It all helps. Develop a strong network of support before the transplant. This will free you up to focus on the patient's needs.

> "One of the hardest things for both of us to learn was to let other people help us. We weren't used to having other people do things for us. We always assumed there would have to be a payback. But people took the kids shopping for school clothes, took them to the show and refused money when I offered it to them. Finally, we had to accept the fact that we could never repay everyone for their kindness. There were too many people helping us for that. It made a big change in our lives to realize how many friends we really had."

Being the Patient's Advocate

Part of being the patient's caregiver is being his or her advocate. Caregivers know information about the patient that doctors and nurses may not have. You may know, for example, how to get your child to do unpleasant tasks. If you are caring for an adult patient, you may know that the patient will be reluctant to ask for pain relief before the pain is severe and more difficult to control.

Although the transplant team works hard to provide the best care for patients, they may not always pick up patient distress signals as easily as a caregiver who knows the patient well. It comforts patients to know that their caregiver is looking out for their well-being only, and is not distracted by the needs of other patients.

> "I saw my job as a gatekeeper — keeping track of details, asking questions, being an advocate for my wife with the

medical staff and taking care of her emotional and physical needs. I was present at all the medical consultations and made sure I paid attention to details like whether she was receiving proper medicines. When visitors came I managed them, depending on whether or not my wife wanted to see them."

Getting Information

Although getting information daily from the patient's doctor is important, it's sometimes hard to accomplish. Find out when the doctors make their rounds each day so you can be there to ask questions. If you can't be present when the doctor visits the patient, find out when you can contact him or her by phone or visit in person.

One family, with multiple caregivers, left a journal with the patient. All caregivers wrote in it daily about the patient's medical care, other important details and feelings. Some people even tape record or videotape meetings with doctors to help keep track of important information.

> "I made a point of becoming very well informed about the transplant process. I felt strongly that I was an advocate for my husband, and in order to be taken seriously and to get the best care for him, I had to be knowledgeable.
>
> At the same time, I worked hard to ignore statistics. They're useful for scientists, but not patients. A person cannot be 20% alive and 80% dead, so it's pointless to get hung up on the numbers."

> "Keep a diary and carry it with you. I would write down everything in it — doctors' instructions, names, phone numbers, maps, etc. One day starts to blend into the next and it becomes impossible to remember everything without taking notes."

Be prepared for the fact that while the patient is hospitalized, the transplant physician who sees the patient daily may change every two-to-four weeks. Find out when doctors rotate, so you can debrief the doctor who is leaving, get some information about the doctor who is about to assume your loved one's care, and prepare the patient for the change.

Flexibility and Patience: Essential Components

As it is with many things in life, each transplant evolves in its own way. There is no way to predict how someone's course will unfold. You'll need to be prepared for ups and downs during the patient's treatment and recovery. Complications can occur, and recovery sometimes takes longer than expected.

After the patient returns home, there can be setbacks. It's not unusual for transplant patients to develop infections and other complications that may require them to be admitted to the hospital.

> "Plan all you can, but expect the unexpected. Plan to be more tired than you can possibly imagine. Take things one day at a time or, if necessary, one hour at a time and hang in there."

> "I tried to say the serenity prayer every day. 'God, grant me the serenity to accept things I cannot change, courage to change the things I can, and the wisdom to know the difference.' "

Keeping a Sense of Humor

Many caregivers say that maintaining a sense of humor, despite the difficulties, helped them and the patient cope.

> "Through all the tears, we managed to find a lot of humor, which kept us all sane. Sometimes things that seem so traumatic at the time can really strike you funny in retrospect. For example, when my sister was having her chemotherapy, the nurses suggested she shave off her hair, rather than let it fall out. My dad wanted to take pictures of it, and we really argued with him about it — it was so upsetting at the time. But a few days later, we all had a good laugh. We couldn't believe we'd been fighting over hair, when there were so many bigger issues at stake."

> "I would rent funny movies or read funny books to my wife. I also found it helpful to share humorous moments with visitors and friends. The transplant was very scary for our friends. My wife and I were in deep denial as we went through it, but our friends understood the severity

of the situation. It made it easier for them to call or visit if we could share some humorous moments with them."

"Pray, cry and talk when you need to, but also keep a positive attitude. During my husband's recovery, we played a lot of cards, talked about all the fun we'd had, and all the fun we were going to have once he was well."

Relaying Information to Others

One task caregivers find hard is keeping family and friends informed about the patient's progress. Relying on friends to help with this task eases the burden. So does relying on technology.

Consider setting up a communication network in advance with family, co-workers and friends.

"It was really draining to get information to all the people who cared. After working all day and being at the hospital, it takes all your energy just to exist some days. My wife and I shared details with four or five close friends who we knew would be a great source of support. For the rest, I recorded a more general message each day on our voicemail."

"My friend's caregiver set up an email list. Each week she sent the entire list an update, including any suggestions she had for supporting the patient at each stage of the process."

Online resources like CaringBridge.org are an excellent way to keep family and friends updated on the patient's progress, and enable them to easily send get-well wishes.

> Each Saturday night, I sent a summary of the week's events to family and friends. I began writing in a journal the day my wife went into the hospital. I spent a half hour each day recording events and our feelings. Initially I did it so my wife would have a record of what happened to her. But it became the way I organized my thoughts, sorted out feelings, and communicated with loved ones. I've continued journaling even to this day.

Know Your Role

Caring for a spouse or partner who is undergoing an autologous transplant is emotionally trying and physically exhausting. Not only do you have to juggle the needs of the patient, your own needs, and those of family members, but you must do it without help from the person with whom you normally share these responsibilities — the patient.

> "I think it's tougher for the caregiver than the patient. The patient can stay focused on getting well, but you also have your normal day-to-day stuff like work, children, bills and other family members to deal with. It's a lot of stress."

To complicate matters, you and the patient may have different ideas about the caregiver's role. You may feel you have to become a medical expert to properly care for the patient, when in reality, what the patient may want most is emotional support.

> "Find out what the patient expects from you. My husband just wanted me there, not to entertain him, but for the feeling of companionship, and to give support and comfort during the long recovery process."

> "It helps to follow the cues from the patient. Do as little or as much as he wants you to do. Help the patient maintain his dignity by letting him take the lead."

Walking the thin line between being an understanding caregiver and wanting the patient to take a more active role in his or her recovery can be difficult. Sometimes caregivers feel that the patient should be making more progress, but don't know how hard to push the issue.

> "Be patient, but also feel your way into becoming more assertive with the patient. I always felt I shouldn't say certain things to my husband, but then I started feeling depressed and isolated. I waited too long to tell him simple things, like he had enough strength to take out the garbage. He became extremely depressed and dependent on me. That was very hard, but eventually we worked things out."

"Getting the patient to bathe, eat, exercise and take medications is not always easy. Sometimes you have to be stern with instructions. Learn to be patient, but kindly persistent. A good caregiver is not a softy."

Changing Relationships

Being the caregiver for a spouse or partner who is recovering from transplant can alter your relationship — at least for a time. The physical and emotional trauma experienced by both the patient and caregiver is often expressed as anger, irritability or depression. In most cases, the problems resolve over time and some eventually share a closer relationship. For others, the changes remain for a long time.

"My husband became very grouchy, impatient and irritable. He expected a lot from me all the time. It was often hard to be patient with him."

"I had to take over all of his responsibilities — paying bills, yard work, etc. Instead of being an equal partner, it was like having another child to worry about. I felt like I'd lost the man I married and just wanted him back."

"We seem to have permanently traded roles. He used to be the more relaxed, practical conscientious partner. Now I have to constantly remind him not to get upset over little things and to be more positive."

"The changes we've noticed are for the better. We made it through one of the most difficult things a couple can go through. It has changed our perspective and led us to make a number of positive changes in our lives. We still fight about nothing from time to time, but our fighting is half-hearted, as though we know it's nothing."

Helping Children Cope

Children of transplant patients share the trauma of their parent's illness and treatment. Depending on their age, they may express their fears in a number of different ways. Some become depressed. Others have behavioral problems, difficulties at school or begin to regress. Still others may worry that they caused or will catch the disease.

For most children, just being separated from their parent for a long period of time is very distressing. Being open and honest with your children about your disease and treatment and allowing them to express their questions and concerns is essential to helping them cope with the experience.

> "Our three children, ages two, seven and eleven, had all kinds of problems. The stress of knowing their mother might not live was overwhelming. I tried to help them by talking with them, over and over again, about my wife's illness. I made sure they understood that there are no stupid questions or feelings."

> "My 13-year-old son became very depressed while his father was undergoing a transplant out of town. In addition to getting him some professional help, I sent him to visit his father over Spring break. It helped him to see his father progressing."

A big concern expressed by our six-year-old daughter was that her mom was going to be bald. We took control of the situation by taking her to the hospital several times before the transplant to see other people and children who were bald.

We then made it a family outing with friends and a movie camera when my wife went to the hair dresser and had her hair buzzed army-style. Our daughter accepted the baldness well and even asked to take her mom to school for 'show and tell'. She was very proud of her bald mom, and my wife went with no reservations.

Coming Home

Everyone looks forward to leaving the hospital or ending the daily visits to the outpatient clinic. Many, however, are unprepared for the fact that for the first months, life at home will not be normal.

In many ways, caring for a transplant patient at home is more difficult than assisting with his or her care while in the hospital or at the outpatient clinic. Medications must be administered, catheters must be carefully cleaned, special diets may have to be followed and infection precautions must be adhered to — all without the help of a readily available nursing staff.

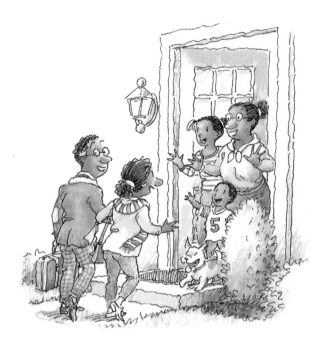

The early weeks and months are often a confusing and stressful time for families. This is a time when many family caregivers experience burnout. Your loved one has survived the rigors of the treatment and you should be happy, but the difficulties are far from over. There are frequent clinic visits, sometimes a hospitalization, and ongoing caregiving responsibilities. Support systems may begin to fall apart as family and friends mistakenly think that life is now back to normal.

> "Picking up the pieces is not easy. For months I felt like I was on autopilot. I forgot how to sleep and constantly felt like I was dragging. There didn't seem to be enough hours in the day or energy in me to take care of everyone's needs. After ten months I wondered, 'When will this be over?' "

It's good to let friends and family members know how they can help. Although some may not be as understanding as you'd like, others will be glad for the opportunity to help and thankful that you are explicit about what you need.

Conclusion

Happily, most people who survive an autologous transplant report that it was worth the difficulties. Caregivers survive, too, although probably changed from the people they were before the experience.

> "Some good came out of this experience, aside from the fact that my daughter is alive. It helped everyone think about what was important in life."

> "I learned a lot about being a caregiver for a seriously ill family member. It has made me (a doctor) and my wife (a nurse) better caregivers for our patients."

Perhaps this three-and-a-half-year-old survivor said it best to his mom about the importance of caregivers:

> "On the first anniversary of his transplant, I told him it was time to visit the clinic again and he asked, 'Why?'

> I said, 'Everyone who took care of you wants to see you and besides, we should thank the doctors for making you better.'

> He looked at me and said, 'No mommy, you made me better.' "

To learn more, go to our website at:

bmtinfonet.org/role-of-caregiver

Autologous Stem Cell Transplants: A Handbook for Patients

Chapter Twelve

PLANNING FOR SURVIVORSHIP

"The transition from being sick to being healthy can be really difficult. There is a tension that exists because you're going back to the life you once knew, but you may not feel like the same person you were before. So, you have to really practice living in the present moment so that your mind doesn't get the best of you."

Melanie Stachelski, 8-year transplant survivor

As a transplant survivor, you have been through an extraordinary experience. As you move forward with your life, you may find yourself feeling different — different from the people around you and different from your former self.

Survivorship may mean a new appreciation of life, new interests or new priorities. It also may mean getting used to side effects and learning to function despite them. Although most of these side effects will resolve by the end of the first year after transplant, some survivors must adjust to side effects long-term.

Transplant survivors find joy in the fact that they have been given a new lease on life. However, protecting your health long-term requires a good understanding of the treatment you've undergone and your risk for developing complications later on. It also requires access to healthcare providers who are knowledgeable about transplantation and its late effects, and can monitor you for complications.

Survivorship Care Plan

Although some patients can return to their transplant center for long-term follow-up care, many cannot. Most primary care physicians and local oncologists have received little or no training in the care of transplant survivors. Thus, you will need a good long-term follow-up plan, prepared by your transplant team, that outlines your medical history, treatments you received and potential long-term issues that may arise, so that your local doctors can provide you with the best care possible.

The symptoms of some complications can resemble other disorders local doctors often see. Without knowledge of your medical background, your local doctor may direct you to specialists or prescribe tests that will miss the actual problem. YOU are an important partner in protecting your health long-term. The more informed you are about your treatment history and risk for long-term complications, the better equipped you will be to advocate for appropriate care.

What Should Be In the Plan?

When you no longer require care at the transplant center, ask your transplant team to prepare a long-term plan for follow-up care that includes the following information:

- the date, dosage and type of chemotherapy you received, including any you received prior to being referred to the transplant center

- the date, type and site of any radiation you received including any you received prior to being referred to the transplant center

- other medications you received while being treated for your disease that have potential long-term health effects

- any serious infections you developed and how they were treated

- if you relapsed after transplant, how it was treated

- potential late effects for each therapy you received including mental health effects

- a list of your medications and allergies

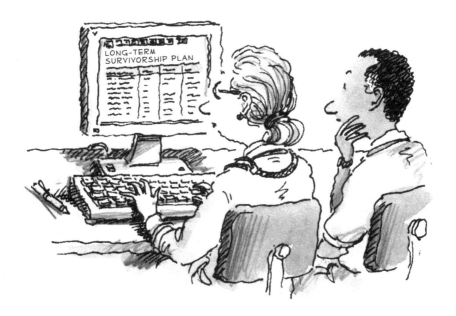

- a list of your vaccinations

- copies of office notes and test results that you can share with your local doctors

- tests and clinical evaluations that should be done periodically to detect possible problems

- whom your doctor should contact for questions and instructions

Make several copies of your long-term follow-up plan and be sure to give it to *all* of your doctors, including dentists. Because you have a complicated medical history, you will need to take responsibility for making sure that all of your doctors know about any medical issues that arise after transplant so that their records are up-to-date. If possible, identify one doctor, physician assistant or nurse practitioner who is willing to coordinate your care so that all the members of your healthcare team are up-to-date on your health history.

Be sure that your transplant team knows the names and contact information for all doctors who are currently caring for you. Update that information annually, particularly if you are changing doctors.

Long-Term Follow-Up Care and Tests

Guidelines for long-term follow-up care have been developed by the Center for International Blood & Marrow Transplant Research (CIBMTR), a leading scientific organization that conducts research on blood stem cell transplantation. The guidelines are written in lay language for patients, and include a summary sheet of tests and periodic exams that you should receive which you can give to each of your doctors.

A link to the guidelines can be found on BMT InfoNet's website at bmtinfonet.org/long-term-health-guidelines.

The Children's Oncology Group has similar guidelines for children who have undergone cancer therapy. These guidelines take into account the effect various chemotherapy drugs and radiation may have on growing children and, thus, include a number of tests and exams not needed by adults. View these guidelines at survivorshipguidelines.org.

Steps you can expect your local doctors to take to protect your health after transplant include:

- tests to evaluate your risk of infection

- redoing your childhood vaccinations six months after transplant, unless your transplant team advises otherwise

- pulmonary function tests to evaluate your lungs, especially if lung abnormalities are present after transplant

- an ophthalmology exam to check your vision and determine whether you are forming cataracts

- annual dental exam to check your teeth and mouth for cavities, dry mouth, gum disease and oral cancer

- annual thyroid function tests

- tests to check your kidney and liver function

- tests to check sex hormone levels

- annual tests to check your heart function

- bone density tests to check for osteoporosis

If the survivor is a child, additional testing will be required to monitor growth, sexual development and learning abilities.

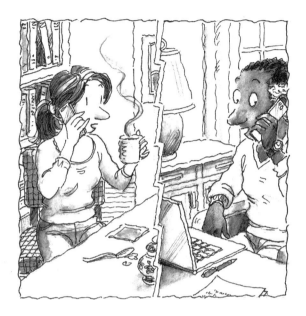

Emotional Well-Being

Emotional distress is common among transplant survivors, at least for a while. It is a significant problem for caregivers as well.

Fear of relapse, changes in body image, a slow rate of recovery, medical setbacks, being socially isolated, financial burdens and not feeling that people really understand what you and your family have been through can create stress even for the most optimistic survivor.

Some survivors find that support groups, online chat rooms or ongoing relationships with other survivors provide the best support.

> "They had a reunion at my transplant center last year and a big patient meeting was held. The first thing you know, someone raised her hand and said, 'Has anyone ever experienced such and such problem?' Well, we were off and running. Somebody else said, 'Do you have memory problems?' I described it differently and other people said, 'Yeah, yeah, that's it.' The meeting was a huge success and we all came out grinning because for the first time we were able to get these issues out on the table and get some

information about them."

Although face-to-face support groups for transplant survivors are rare, there are online support groups and telephone support programs that many survivors find helpful. BMT InfoNet's Caring Connections Program links patients and family members with others who have been through transplant and can provide support. You can request a connection at bmtinfonet.org/caring-connection or by phoning 888-597-7674.

There are many Facebook and other online groups where transplant survivors can connect. You can "like" BMT InfoNet's Bone Marrow and Stem Cell Transplant Club on Facebook, or join our closed Facebook group BMT InfoNet Celebrating a 2nd Chance at Life.

The services of a psychiatrist, psychologist, social worker or other counselor help some survivors get back a sense of well-being.

> "Fifteen months later when I ended the counseling sessions, I thanked the psychiatrist and told him, 'My transplant doctor gave me back my life, but you put the quality back in my life.'"

Some survivors experience survivor guilt. It may happen when another transplant patient they know relapses or does not survive the transplant. Support groups, counseling and clergy can be good resources to help manage these feelings.

Fear of relapse is a major concern, particularly during the early years after transplant. It may take a long time before you are able to make long-term plans or spend a day without thinking about your disease or treatment.

Changing Relationships with Family Members

Marriages often change after transplant. Some couples report that their relationship is the same or better than before the transplant. For others the opposite is true.

> "Going through the transplant strengthened our marital relationship. We threw out all the trash that had accumulated over the years and got our priorities straight."

"After my transplant, I changed in ways that my wife could not understand. I wanted to go a million miles an hour and experience everything. Activities and friends that were now very important to me seemed trivial to her. Our marriage finally ended in divorce last fall."

"The whole experience frightened my husband no end. You don't realize how hard it is on the spouse until it's over. He doesn't want to talk about it, think about it or hear about it. I couldn't even get him to congratulate me on my transplant anniversary. Don't get me wrong, he's a great guy and we love each other very much. But it would be nice to be able to talk with him about the experience."

Relationships with children can also change after transplant.

"The transplant was very hard on my daughters who were sixteen, thirteen and two at the time. They were terrified of losing their mother, and each of them showed their stress in a different way. The oldest felt responsible for the younger two if I died, and that was a big burden for someone her age. Even after I came home, my middle one was afraid that I would be sick again, and didn't know how to talk about her fears. The little one literally clung to me for two years. Working through these problems was a long ordeal, but they've all grown to be very mature, responsible kids. I'm very proud of them and they're proud of me."

A family therapist may be able to help you work through strained relationships and enable each party to understand the other's perspective. Keeping the lines of communication open is key.

The Bottom Line

It may take a while before the constant worrying about your health is over for both you and your loved ones. While physical well-being is important, strong family relationships, friendships, inner spirituality and helping others are also important factors that make for a good quality of life. Many survivors feel the transplant experience helped them get their priorities straight and prompted them to live each day to the fullest, rather than put off the important things for the future.

Some say the experience taught them a lot about what their bodies and minds are capable of doing. Prior to the transplant, everyone is frightened of potential physical complications and pain, and most survivors experience emotional ups and downs for many months following the transplant. Yet, they find ways to cope with these problems and enjoy their second chance at life.

"It took almost two years for me to adjust and reshape my life. It required counseling, support group meetings, constant family support, the loyalty and help from friends and a renewed faith in God. I am now a reasonably happy and content survivor. I've gained peace of mind and peace of soul. I'm finally getting a glimpse of who I really am, and I like what I'm seeing. I still have lingering complications, but if I never feel any better physically than I do right now, I'll still count my blessings. The transplant was, indeed, a traumatic experience, but it gave me the only chance I had to live, and I'm glad that I took it."

For more on long-term health guidelines, go to

bmtinfonet.org/long-term-health-guidelines

Chapter Thirteen

LATE EFFECTS OF TRANSPLANT

The bone marrow transplant affected my life in every way. I am thankful to wake up each morning. I have learned compassion and empathy for those unable to be 'normal'. I have learned how much it means when others are kind. I have learned the value of a family in my life. I have had a paper on my refrigerator for the last five years that reads, 'My goal is to live forever, so far, so good.' The seasons change on our Iowa farm, the crops and animals grow. I, too, hope to keep changing and growing.
Kathleen Jones, 22-year survivor of two transplants

Some of the complications associated with a stem cell transplant are not apparent until several months, or even years after treatment. Most of them resolve with time, but others may be permanent and need attention long-term.

Late effects of transplant may include:

- attention and memory problems

- chronic fatigue and difficulty sleeping

- eye problems

- bone loss

- peripheral neuropathy (numbness and tingling in hands and feet)

- kidney, lung or heart issues

- sexual difficulties

- infertility

- secondary cancers

- relapse

Children may experience additional problems with growth, pubertal development, and early onset heart problems.

> No one experiences all of these complications. Your risk for developing problems after transplant will depend on your disease, the amount and type of chemotherapy and radiation you had, your age and prior treatment history. Many complications can be prevented with proper screening and prompt treatment.

Attention and Memory Problems

For many patients, a surprising side effect of transplant is a change in the way they process information. These changes are called cognitive changes and can be very frustrating for both the survivor and family caregiver.

In some patients the changes are very subtle; in others they are more severe.

You may experience:

- memory lapses

- trouble concentrating

- difficulty multitasking

- problems with organization

- difficulty remembering words during a conversation

These problems usually diminish or completely resolve over time, but some patients continue to experience cognitive issues long-term. Consult a neurologist if the problem persists. There are a variety of strategies you can use to function well despite the changes. Go to bmtinfonet.org/cognitive for tips on how to manage cognitive problems.

Chronic Fatigue

Chronic fatigue is a common complaint following transplant. It can interfere with mood, physical activity, job performance and sleep.

Unlike the fatigue most people experience in everyday life, rest does not always relieve it.

Fatigue can be caused by a number of factors including:

- anemia

- depression

- pain

- sleep disorders

- electrolyte imbalances

- infection

- poorly functioning immune system

- thyroid disorder or other hormone deficiencies

- adrenal insufficiency

- malnutrition

- dehydration

- lack of exercise which leads to deconditioning

- stress

- medications that act on the brain and spinal cord

- inflammatory agents such as IL-6, cytokines and interferons

Survivors who experience fatigue after transplant often complain about decreased energy, a generalized weakness and/or decreased motivation. Fatigue can cause sadness, frustration and irritability. It can make it difficult to perform daily tasks and affect memory.

Be sure to report chronic fatigue to your healthcare team. There are tests that can be performed to check for possible causes like anemia or thyroid problems which are easily treated.

Drinking sufficient liquids and consuming enough carbohydrates and protein are important tools in managing fatigue. Your transplant team can refer you to a nutritionist who can help develop a plan tailored to your needs.

Conserve your energy for the times of the day that you need it most. Sit down when bathing or preparing meals. Plan to do necessary activities at the time of day when you have the most energy. Pace yourself, avoid rushing and delegate responsibilities when possible.

A number of medications can help with temporary fatigue. These include Provigil®, Nuvigil®, Ritalin® and Adderall®. Cognitive behavioral therapy can also help manage fatigue. Learn more about managing chronic fatigue at bmtinfonet. org/fatigue-and-sleep.

> Exercise and physical activity can improve symptoms of fatigue. Even five-to-ten minutes of exercise several times daily can help. Consider enrolling in an exercise class at a gym or local yoga studio to maintain a schedule of physical exercise.

If fatigue interferes with your ability to work, consider talking with your employer about alternate ways to manage your workload. Set realistic goals, perhaps shorten your hours or request a disability leave of absence.

Don't be embarrassed to ask for help. TriageCancer.org/employment has excellent information about employment rights that you may find helpful.

Difficulty Sleeping

Sleep problems are common among transplant survivors, as well as family caregivers, and can persist for years. Insufficient sleep over a long period of time can create serious health problems such as heart disease, diabetes and obesity. Poor sleep can also contribute to:

- headaches
- daytime fatigue
- depression
- anxiety
- substance abuse
- attention, concentration and memory problems
- irritability

Cognitive behavioral therapy for insomnia (CBT-I) helps patients understand their sleep, and change the thoughts and behaviors that interfere with sleep. In six-to-eight sessions, a therapist who specializes in CBT-I can help you:

- track and understand your current sleep behavior

- identify behaviors that interfere with sleep

- adopt habits that promote a good night's rest

- become aware of negative thoughts that make sleep problems worse

> Doctors often prescribe sleep medication for sleep problems. However, you may also be able to achieve a good night's rest using cognitive behavioral therapy designed specifically for insomnia (CBT-I). In fact, the American College of Physicians recommends that all adult patients receive cognitive behavioral therapy for insomnia as the initial treatment, rather than medication.

Sleep-promoting habits that a therapist might help you develop include:

- establishing a regular sleep schedule. It's especially important to wake up at the same time each day, including weekends.

- using your bed only for sleep and sex. This helps train your body to recognize your bed for these purposes only.

- getting out of bed at night, rather than laying awake, if you are having trouble falling asleep

- prior to bedtime, making a list of things you need to do the next day, so you don't stay awake worrying if you will remember them

You can find a trained sleep therapist through the Society for Behavioral Sleep Medicine at behavioralsleep.org or by phoning 859-312-8880. If none exists in your area, try these print resources:

- Overcoming Insomnia, by Jack D. Edinger and Colleen E. Carney

- The Insomnia Workbook, by Stephanie A. Silberman, PhD, DABSM

- Say Good Night to Insomnia, by Gregg D. Jacobs, PhD

There are also online cognitive behavioral therapy programs for people with sleep issues such a myshut*i*.com and sleepio.com. These programs are available to people whose employer has signed up for the service, or you can volunteer to be part of one of their clinical trials.

Eyes

Cataracts are a common side effect of transplant. If you develop a cataract, it can be surgically removed in an outpatient setting.

If you had total body irradiation, you may experience dry eyes after transplant. The problem can usually be managed with artificial tears or ointments.

Bone Loss

Loss of bone density (osteoporosis) sometimes occurs after transplant. It is most common in people who are:

- female
- older
- menopausal
- inactive
- have a small frame
- treated with steroids

If your bone density is low, your doctor may recommend:

- exercise
- calcium
- vitamin D
- hormone replacement therapy
- bisphosphonate

Avascular necrosis (joint deterioration) occurs in five-to-ten percent of transplant survivors, particularly those exposed to high dosages of steroids over a prolonged period of time. It usually affects the hips, but can occur in the shoulder and ankles as well. Surgery is often used to correct the problem. Many transplant centers now routinely measure calcium and vitamin D levels in the first year after transplant and adjust supplements as needed.

Kidneys

Kidney disease can occur following transplant. The risk of kidney disease is greatest among patients who have multiple myeloma and those who were treated with total body irradiation.

Treatment for kidney disease varies depending on the particular type of kidney problem you have. If you have kidney problems, be sure to talk with your doctor about all medications you take, including herbal supplements, as some can make the problem worse.

Lungs

Some chemotherapies, such as bleomycin, carmustine (BiCNU®) and brentuximab (Adcetris®), as well as radiation, can cause scarring in the lungs. Radiation and surgery to remove infections can affect breathing as well.

Think of exercise as a "vital sign" and report any changes in exercise tolerance to your doctor. Your doctor may order tests to determine changes in lung function.

Avoid smoking, including e-cigarettes, and limit your exposure to vapors in the workplace.

Heart

Some transplant survivors have a slightly increased risk of a heart attack or congestive heart failure. Risk factors include:

- radiation to the chest (not total body irradiation)

- hormonal changes

- drugs such as cyclophosphamide (Cytoxan®), melphalan (Alkeran® or Evomela®) and anthracyclines

To protect you heart, have regular check-ups for blood pressure, diabetes and cholesterol. Exercise regularly and report any health changes to your doctor.

Peripheral Neuropathy

Peripheral neuropathy is a nerve condition that sometimes occurs after transplant. Peripheral neuropathy can cause pain or tingling in the hands and feet. The discomfort may be greater at night or in cold weather.

Some drugs used during or after transplant can cause peripheral neuropathy. These include:

- cisplatin
- vincristine
- thalidomide (THALOMID®)
- lenalidomide (REVLIMID®)
- bortezomib (VELCADE®)

To learn how pain from neuropathy is managed, go to Chapter 10, Relieving Pain.

Dental Problems

Decreased saliva production may occur after transplant and can increase the risk of tooth decay and gum disease. Prescription toothpastes with high fluoride content, such as Prevident®, or fluoride rinses provided by your dentist may help prevent these complications. Frequent follow-up with a dentist is important to prevent serious dental issues.

Fertility and Sexual Health

Most, but not all, transplant survivors will be infertile after transplant, especially those who received cyclophosphamide (Cytoxan®) or total body irradiation as part of the conditioning regimen. (For more on infertility and options for creating a family after transplant see Chapter Fifteen, Family Planning.)

Sexual difficulties are common after transplant, but are often not discussed by patients and physicians. Physical as well as psychological factors can contribute to problems with intimacy after transplant. (See Chapter Fourteen, Sexual Health after Transplant for a more detailed discussion.)

Secondary Cancers

A small percentage of transplant survivors are at risk for developing a new cancer several years after treatment. The most common types of cancer seen are acute myelogenous leukemia, skin cancer, breast cancer and mouth cancer.

Regular check-ups for signs of these cancers are important. Your transplant team can advise you whether you are at risk for developing a second cancer.

Relapse

Sometimes a patient's disease comes back after transplant. This is called relapse.

For some, relapse is an expected event. Multiple myeloma patients, for example, know that their disease will eventually return. For them, the objective of transplant is to slow the progression of their disease and extend their life.

Some patients are put on maintenance therapy after a transplant to reduce the risk of or delay relapse.

If you relapse after transplant, your doctor can advise you on available treatment options. A second transplant, either with your own cells or donor cells, may be an option. You may be eligible for a clinical trial testing new drugs or therapies.

Thoroughly examine your options so you can make a choice that is right for you. Don't be afraid to get a second opinion. Different institutions may have different treatment options to offer you.

Late Effects in Children

Growth Problems

Some children experience slow or stunted growth after transplant. The problem occurs most often in children who received total body irradiation.

If your child was age ten or less at the time of transplant, growth hormone replacement therapy may help spur growth. Growth hormone therapy does not typically improve height in children who were older than ten at the time of transplant.

A thyroid hormone deficiency can also affect your child's growth and may not show up until two or more years after transplant. Your child should be tested regularly to ensure that this is not an issue.

Learning and Organizational Challenges

Many children who have had a transplant excel in school with no problems. However, some children experience learning difficulties after transplant and will need special accommodations at school.

Learning problems are more common among children transplanted at an early age and those who had total body irradiation. Problems may include:

- difficulty remembering things
- poor eye-hand coordination
- problem solving difficulties
- difficulty sustaining attention
- organizational problems

A pediatric neuropsychologist can test your child for learning disabilities and help you obtain any necessary accommodations your child may need at school to succeed academically. Similar tests help teens and young adults identify professions that match their learning and performance skills.

Puberty and Fertility

Most girls who are transplanted during or after puberty experience ovarian failure or premature menopause and will be infertile.

If your child retains her fertility after transplant, she may have a higher than normal risk of problems during pregnancy. However, infants born to women who had a transplant as a child are as healthy as those born to women who did not have a transplant.

Boys who are transplanted before puberty typically maintain normal testosterone levels. However most boys, regardless of age, will be infertile. If your child retains his fertility, his offspring will not have a higher risk of health problems than the general population.

Dental Problems

Children transplanted before the age of five may experience dental problems, such as loose teeth, tooth loss and dry mouth and may be unable to wear braces. It is important that your child be followed by a dentist who is experienced in treating children who've undergone high-dose chemotherapy or total body irradiation.

Heart Problems

Some chemotherapy drugs used prior to transplant, such as doxorubicin (Adriamycin®), daunorubicin (Cerubidine®) and mitoxantrone, can damage a child's heart muscle cells. Total body irradiation can also increase the risk of heart problems later in your child's life.

Although there may be no symptoms of a heart problem for several years, your child should have an echocardiogram every one-to-five years to monitor for heart problems.

Take Charge of Your Health

Your autologous transplant has given you a new lease on life. Protecting your health requires a life-long commitment to regular check-ups, reporting new problems to your doctors, and being persistent in getting the care you need to address any health issues.

Lifestyle changes can make a big difference in your long-term quality of life. Regular exercise, a good diet and limiting the stress in your life can help you make the most of your second chance at life.

Learn more about potential late complications after transplant at:

bmtinfonet.org/late-effects

Chapter Fourteen

SEXUAL HEALTH AFTER TRANSPLANT

No one ever mentioned that my sex life might be affected by transplant. It wouldn't have changed my decision to have a transplant, but it sure would have prepared me better for what to expect and what to do about it.

Robert W, 16-year transplant survivor

It's the elephant in the room: sexual difficulties after transplant. No one talks about it upfront, especially when life and death matters are of primary concern.

Although pop culture is full of sexy images and dialogue, frank and honest discussion about sex is not something that is encouraged. Many people feel embarrassed to even bring it up with their doctor and physicians are equally uncomfortable discussing it with patients. Hence, the topic is often not addressed and patients suffer in silence.

But changes in sexuality after transplant are common, and knowing what to expect and how to deal with these changes can ease distress between partners.

Not everyone experiences changes in sexuality after transplant. However, in one study, 46% percent of men and 80% percent of women reported lower sexual activity and sexual function five years after transplant than those who had not had a transplant. Women who resumed sexual relations during the first year after transplant appeared to have less difficulty later than those who did not.

Both radiation and chemotherapy can affect sexual function after transplant. Depression, mood changes, some antidepressants and pain medicines can also affect sexual relations.

Changes in sexuality come as a surprise for both patient and partner alike. Fortunately, if sexual difficulties do arise there are several things you can try to remedy the situation and make sexual relationships pleasurable once again.

Talk openly with your partner about any changes in desire, arousal or sexual satisfaction that you are experiencing. You will need to work together to address the problem, and communicating about these issues will help you develop a plan. The solution may mean changing the way you seek and enjoy intimate relations. A consultation with a trained sex therapist can be helpful in identifying ways to regain intimacy.

Males

Men who undergo total body irradiation may experience damage to the small blood vessels in the penis. This can make it difficult to achieve an erection. Radiation and some types of high-dose chemotherapy can cause nerve damage and reduce testosterone levels, which can decrease desire.

Difficulty achieving an erection can be treated by medications such as Viagra®, Cialis® or Levitra®. These drugs relax smooth muscle cells that let blood flow into the penis. However, they don't work as well if nerves have been damaged and they do not increase desire.

Injections of drugs such as Caverject® and Edex® can help men achieve erections. Vacuum devices, although cumbersome, are also very helpful.

Talk with your doctor about whether these or other therapies, such as surgical implants, are appropriate for you.

Most men recover normal testosterone levels between six months and two years after transplant. For those who continue to have low or low-normal testosterone levels, testosterone replacement can help.

Females

Total body irradiation and high-dose chemotherapy usually cause premature ovarian failure. Ovarian failure makes it harder for the vagina to stretch and reduces the lubricating fluid in the vagina. The vaginal skin becomes thin and fragile. During intercourse there can be bleeding, soreness or burning. This pain, as well as the usual menopausal symptoms like hot flashes and reduced testosterone, can reduce a woman's desire for sexual intercourse.

Many women report decreased physical arousal, difficulty reaching orgasm or orgasms that are not as intense as they were before transplant. Vaginal moisturizers such as Replens®, KY Liquibeads™ or similar products used regularly can be useful. Water or silicon-based lubricants specifically designed for use before intercourse can also help. Some women find that a vaginal dilator improves blood flow to and elasticity of the vagina.

Many women experience early menopause following transplant. Hormone replacement therapy can be useful, although it has been controversial in recent years. A discussion with your doctor about the risks and benefits of this therapy will help you decide whether it is right for you.

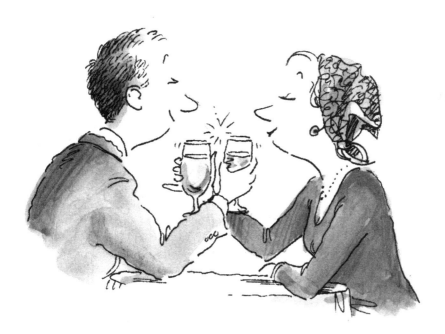

Psychological Issues

Aside from the physical difficulties created by transplant, psychological issues can also affect your sexual desire and pleasure. Both you and your partner may worry about infection, particularly if your immune system has not fully recovered. Weight loss or weight gain, scars, temporary hair loss and other physical changes can affect how you feel about your body and sexual appeal.

Some people find that taking it slow and easy helps them transition back into a satisfactory sexual relationship. There are a variety of different techniques you can use to achieve intimacy with a partner. A sex therapist can help you identify some new techniques to try.

The most important thing is to maintain honest, open communication with your partner about what both of you need and can achieve. Don't assume you know what your partner wants. You need to ask. Make a plan and set some ground rules. This can eliminate frustration and misunderstanding and speed sexual recovery.

Resources

To get a referral to a certified sex therapist in your area contact the American Association of Sexuality Educators, Counselors and Therapists at aasect.org or phone 202-449-1099.

Will2Love.com is an online resource designed to help cancer survivors regain sexual health after transplant.

To learn more, go to our website at:

bmtinfonet.org/sexual-health-after-transplant

Chapter Fifteen

FAMILY PLANNING

Deciding to undergo a transplant was the hardest decision of my life. The odds of survival were not in my favor, and the fact that I would be infertile after the transplant tore me apart. I finally decided I had too much to live for, and too much more to accomplish to give up. I agreed to have the transplant.

Lisa Powell, 7-year transplant survivor

Most, but not all, patients who undergo an autologous transplant will be infertile afterward. The likelihood of infertility depends on your age, gender, sexual maturity and the type and amount of chemotherapy and/or radiation you received as part of the conditioning regimen.

Fortunately, there are options available if you wish to have children after transplant. Medically assisted reproduction techniques such as artificial insemination and in-vitro fertilization are options for women. Sperm banking before transplant may enable men to have children after transplant. Adoption is another option.

Understanding the options in advance of your transplant will enable you to better plan for children after transplant and relieve some of the stress associated with the prospect of infertility.

Medically Assisted Reproduction

Couples who wish to bear children after transplant may be helped by medically assisted reproduction technology. While not always successful, assisted reproduction allows women who are infertile to bear children, and men to contribute to the genetic make-up of their child.

Artificial Insemination

Artificial insemination is a procedure in which sperm are injected into a woman's vagina at the point in her monthly cycle when mature eggs are most likely to be fertilized. If the sperm fertilizes an egg and the resulting embryo implants in the lining of the uterus, a pregnancy begins.

Frozen sperm have been successfully used in artificial insemination. Thus, if you are facing the possibility of infertility after transplant, you may wish to bank some of your sperm prior to transplant.

Sperm banking is a relatively simple procedure. Several samples of sperm are collected over a one-to-three week period and cryopreserved (frozen at very low temperatures) in sterile containers. If your sperm count is lower due to illness or prior chemotherapy, it may still be possible to collect enough sperm for future use.

If your sperm is not frozen prior to transplant, it may be possible for you and your partner to have a child using donor sperm. A donor may be someone you know or sperm from a sperm bank.

For men who have a very low sperm count or low sperm motility after transplant, intracytoplasmic sperm injection (ICSI) may be a treatment option. In this procedure, a reproductive specialist inserts a single sperm into the egg to fertilize it. The egg is then implanted in the woman's uterus.

In-Vitro Fertilization

Women who are infertile after transplant may be able to carry a child to term with the help of in-vitro fertilization (IVF). IVF enables eggs to be fertilized by sperm in a laboratory dish. The resulting embryos are then transferred to the woman's uterus. If an embryo implants in the uterine lining, a pregnancy begins.

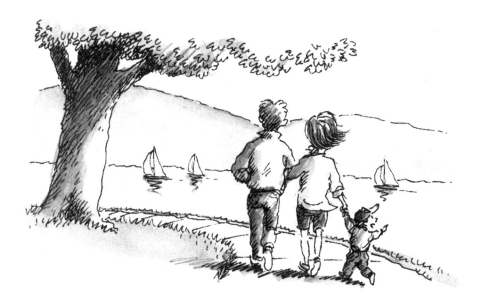

IVF can be done using your own eggs that were collected before transplant or eggs donated by a friend, relative or anonymous donor. Although in-vitro fertilization with donated eggs does not allow you to contribute to the genetic make-up of your child, you can carry and nurture a child in your womb during pregnancy and mother it thereafter.

If you are considering having your own eggs stored prior to your transplant, you should first consult your transplant physician. Some of the drugs used to stimulate egg production might accelerate the disease or otherwise interfere with treatment. In some cases, there may not be sufficient time to complete the procedure before transplant.

New alternatives for preserving fertility before transplant are being explored. Several investigators are exploring whether removing an entire ovary and freezing the outer layer that contains the eggs for future use is a viable option.

In-vitro fertilization is expensive, and insurance may or may not cover the cost. It can take several cycles before in-vitro fertilization is successful, and some couples may not be successful at all. Nonetheless, several transplant survivors have succeeded in becoming pregnant after transplant with the help of in-vitro fertilization.

To learn more about assisted reproduction techniques contact:

LIVESTRONG Fertility
855-220-7777
livestrong.org/we-can-help/fertility-services

American Society for Reproductive Medicine
205-978-5000
asrm.org

Oncofertility Consortium
866-708-3378
oncofertility.northwestern.edu

Adoption

After transplant, you may find it difficult to adopt a child in the U.S. through a traditional adoption agency. Most adoption agencies have strict requirements about the health history of adopting parents and may deny you because of your prior illness and treatment.

However, it may be possible to arrange for a private adoption. Hiring a skilled adoption attorney to help you is wise. Your attorney can prevent you from making costly mistakes, tell you what is allowed under State law and provide advice on how to publicize your interest in adopting a child. You can find a reputable attorney that specializes in adoption law by contacting the Academy of Adoption & Assisted Reproduction Attorneys at 317-407-8422 or visit their website adoptionart.org.

Adopting a child from a country other than the U.S. is another option to consider. Each country has its own guidelines regarding the adopting parents' health history, which may be less restrictive than those of U.S. adoption agencies.

Many transplant survivors have successfully adopted children after transplant and are enjoying their role as a parent to the fullest.

> "It wasn't until a couple of years after my transplant that we got into the adoption process. I was concerned about disclosing my cancer diagnosis because it could have scared some birth parents off. But I know for a fact that my child's birth parents actually chose us *because* of my

cancer history. They saw us as resilient, having gone through so much, and understood that we couldn't have children of our own.

Adoption was not how I envisioned building a family, but I could not ask for two more precious children."

To learn more about adoption options go to:

Child Welfare Information Gateway
800-394-3366
childwelfare.gov

North American Council on Adoptable Children
651-644-3036
nacac.org

To learn more, go to our website at:

bmtinfonet.org/build-family-after-transplant

ABOUT BLOOD CELLS

Blood is composed of many different kinds of cells, each with a specific function. Most blood cells are formed in the bone marrow and released into the bloodstream at various stages of maturity. In healthy adults, an estimated 500 million new blood cells are produced each hour.

During your treatment, the medical team will be monitoring the level of various types of blood cells. Those that you will hear about most often are red blood cells, white blood cells and platelets.

Red blood cells (erythrocytes) pick up oxygen in the lungs and transport it to tissues throughout the body. They also pick up carbon dioxide from tissues and transport it back to the lungs where it is exhaled.

White blood cells (leukocytes) are needed to fight infection. The main types of white blood cells and their functions are described on the next page.

Platelets (thrombocytes) are the smallest cell elements in the bloodstream. Platelets are needed to control bleeding.

All blood cells evolve from primitive cells in the marrow called pluripotent stem cells. Pluripotent stem cells are unique cells that can replicate themselves as well as produce two other types of stem cells called myeloid stem cells and lymphoid stem cells. These stem cells, in turn, either replicate themselves or produce other cells that eventually evolve into blood cells. A group of white blood cells called lymphocytes evolve from lymphoid stem cells. Red blood cells, platelets and other types of white blood cells evolve from the myeloid stem cell.

White Blood Cells

There are five main types of white blood cells: lymphocytes, monocytes, neutrophils, eosinophils and basophils.

Lymphocytes are the smallest white blood cells. Lymphocytes fight viral infections and help destroy bacteria, fungi and other parasites. One type of lymphocyte, the T-cell, is the body's main defense against viruses and protozoa. A second type, the B-cell, produces proteins called antibodies. The antibodies attach to the surface of foreign organisms or the cells they've invaded. They then summon another group of proteins, called complement, to surround the organism or infected cell and dissolve a hole in it.

Monocytes are the largest white blood cells. They can surround and destroy invading bacteria and fungi. They also clean up the debris that is left after other white blood cells destroy foreign organisms. When monocytes leave the bloodstream and enter tissues or organs, they can evolve into larger cells called macrophages. Macrophages have an even greater ability to destroy foreign organisms that invade the body.

Neutrophils (also called granulocytes) fight bacterial infections. They patrol the body via the blood stream or lymph system, and destroy harmful bacteria. (The lymph system is a network of vessels that run alongside the blood stream.)

Eosinophils attack protozoa that cause infection.

Basophils are the least common type of white blood cell and their function is not completely understood. They play an important role in regulating allergic reactions such as asthma, hives, hay fever and reactions to drugs.

Blast Cells

White blood cells pass through several stages of development before maturing into lymphocytes, monocytes, neutrophils, eosinophils or basophils. Very immature white blood cells are called blast cells or blasts.

Blast cells are usually found only in the bone marrow. If a large number of blast cells are detected in the bloodstream, the patient most likely has leukemia. A smaller number of blasts are sometimes detected in the bloodstream of patients who are recovering from chemotherapy or an infection. This is common and is *not* an indication that the patient has leukemia.

UNDERSTANDING BLOOD TESTS

Have you ever wondered what all those blood tests were measuring? Here's a guide to help you make sense of the results.

Complete Blood Count (CBC)
Describes the number, type and form of each blood cell. It includes all tests described below.

Red Blood Cell Count (RBC)
Counts the number of red blood cells in a single drop (a microliter) of blood. Normal ranges vary according to age and sex.

    Men: 4.5 to 6.2 million
    Women: 4.2 to 5.4 million
    Children: 4.6 to 4.8 million

A low RBC count may indicate anemia, excess body fluid or hemorrhaging. A high RBC count may indicate polycythemia (an excessive number of red blood cells in the blood) or dehydration.

Total Hemoglobin Concentration
Hemoglobin gives red blood cells their color and carries oxygen from the lungs to cells. This test measures grams of hemoglobin in a

deciliter (100 ml) of blood, which can help physicians determine the severity of anemia or polycythemia.

Normal values are:

Men:	14 to 18 g/dL
Women:	12 to 16 g/dL
Children:	11 to 13 g/dL

A significant anemia occurs when the hemoglobin drops below 7-8 g/dL.

Hematocrit

Hematocrit measures the percentage of red blood cells in the sample. Normal values vary greatly:

Men:	45% to 57%
Women:	37% to 47%
Children:	36% to 40%

Erythrocyte (RBC) Indices

Three indices that measure the size of red blood cells and amount of hemoglobin contained in each. Mean corpuscular volume (MCV) measures the volume of red blood cells. Normal is 84 to 99 fl. Mean corpuscular hemoglobin (MCH) measures the amount of hemoglobin in an average cell. Normal is 26 to 32 pg. Mean corpuscular hemoglobin concentration (MCHC) measures the concentration of hemoglobin in red blood cells. Normal is 30% to 36%.

White Blood Cell Count (WBC)

Measures the number of white blood cells in a drop (microliter) of blood. Normal values range from 4,100 to 10,900 but can be altered greatly by factors such as exercise, stress and disease. A low WBC may indicate viral infection or toxic reaction. A high WBC count may indicate infection, leukemia, or tissue damage. An increased risk of infection occurs once the WBC drops below 1,000/microliter, and especially below 500/microliter.

WBC Differential

Determines the percentage of each type of white blood cell in the sample. Multiplying the percentage by the total count of white blood cells indicates the actual number of each type of white blood cell in the sample. Normal values are:

Type	Percentage	Number
Neutrophil	50-60%	3,000-7,000/microliter
Eosinophils	1-4%	50-400
Basophils	0.5-2%	25-100
Lymphocytes	20-40%	1,000-4,000
Monocytes	2-9%	100-600

A serious infection can develop once the total neutrophil count (percentage of neutrophils times total WBC) drops below 500/microliter.

Platelet Count

Measures the number of platelets in a drop (microliter) of blood. Platelet counts increase during strenuous activity and in certain conditions called myeloproliferative disorders. Infections, inflammations, malignancies and removal of the spleen can also cause platelet counts to increase. Platelet counts decrease just before menstruation. Normal values range from 150,000 to 400,000 per microliter. A count below 50,000 can result in spontaneous bleeding; below 10,000, patients are at risk of severe, life-threatening bleeding.

Autologous Stem Cell Transplants: A Handbook for Patients

GLOSSARY OF TERMS

This glossary contains terms and abbreviations you may encounter during your treatment that are not explained elsewhere in this book.

ABW: Actual body weight.

Acute: Having severe symptoms and a short course.

Adjuvant therapy: Additional drug or other treatment designed to enhance the effectiveness of the primary treatment.

ADR: Adverse drug reaction.

ALC: Absolute lymphocyte count.

Alkaline phosphatase: An enzyme produced by the liver or bone.

Allergen: Any substance that causes an allergy.

Allergy: An inappropriate and harmful response of the immune system to normally harmless substances.

Alopecia: Loss of hair.

AML: Acute myeloid leukemia or acute myelogenous leukemia.

Anaphylaxis: Acute allergic reaction that causes shortness of breath, rash, wheezing, hypotension.

Anaphylactic shock: A life-threatening allergic reaction characterized by a swelling of body tissues including the throat, difficulty in breathing, and a sudden fall in blood pressure.

ANC: Absolute neutrophil count.

Anemia: Too few red blood cells in the bloodstream, resulting in insufficient oxygen to tissues and organs.

Anorexia: Loss of appetite.

Antibiotic: A drug used to fight bacterial infections.

Antibody: A protein produced by the body, in response to the pres-ence of a foreign substance, that fights the invading organism.

Antiemetic: A drug used to control nausea and vomiting.

Antigen: A substance that evokes a response from the body's immune system resulting in the production of antibodies or other defensive action by white blood cells.

Antiserum: Serum that contains antibodies.

Antitoxins: Antibodies that inactivate toxins produced by certain bacteria.

Apheresis: A procedure by which blood is withdrawn from a patient's arm and circulated through a machine that removes certain components and returns the remaining components to the patient. This procedure is used to remove platelets from platelet donors' blood, or stem cells from patients undergoing a stem cell harvest.

Aplasia: A failure to develop or form. In bone marrow aplasia, the marrow cavity is empty.

Ascites: Accumulation of fluid in the stomach area.

Ataxia: Loss of balance.

Autoantibody: An antibody that reacts against a person's own tissue.

Autograft: Bone marrow or stem cells removed from the patient to be used in an autologous transplant.

Autoimmune disease: A disease that results when the immune system attacks the body's own tissues.

Baseline test: Test that measures an organ's normal level of functioning. Used to determine if any changes in organ function occur following treatment.

Biological response modifiers: Substances, either natural or man-made, that boost, direct, or restore normal immune defenses.

Biopsy: Removal of tissue for examination under a microscope, to enable the doctor to make a proper diagnosis.

BM: Bone marrow.

BMSC: Bone marrow stem cell.

BMT: Bone marrow transplant. Also used as an abbreviation for blood and marrow transplant.

BRM: Biological response modifier.

Calorie: A measure of energy your body gets from food.

Carbohydrate: One of the three nutrients that supply calories to the body.

Cardiac: Pertaining to the heart.

Catheter: Small, flexible plastic tube inserted into a portion of the body to administer or remove fluids.

CBSC: Cord blood stem cell.

Central line: Central venous catheter.

Central venous catheter: Small, flexible plastic tube inserted into the large vein above the heart, through which drugs and blood products can be given, and blood samples withdrawn.

Chemo: Chemotherapy.

Chemo-responsive: Responds to chemotherapy. For example, a tumor is chemo-responsive if it shrinks in size following chemotherapy.

Chemotherapy: Drug or combination of drugs designed to kill cancerous cells.

Chromosomes: Physical structures in the cell's nucleus that house the genes. Each human cell has 23 pairs of chromosomes.

Chronic: Persisting for a long time.

CNS: Central nervous system.

Conjunctivitis: Eye inflammation.

CP: Chronic phase.

CPR: Cardio pulmonary resuscitation.

CR: Complete remission.

Cryopreservation: To preserve by freezing at very low temperatures.

CSF: Colony stimulating factor.

CT scan: Also called a CAT scan or CT-X-ray. A three-dimensional x-ray.

Cytogenetic remission: (see Remission, cytogenetic.)

Cytokines: Powerful chemical substances secreted by cells. They play an important role in regulating the immune system.

DC: Dendritic cell.

Dendritic: Rare but important cells that spur T-cells into action.

Dermatitis: A skin rash.

DFS: Disease free survival.

DNA (deoxyribonucleic acid): Nucleic acid that is found in the cell nucleus and that is the carrier of genetic information.

Dysgeusia: Changes in the way foods are perceived to taste.

Dysphasia: Difficulty swallowing.

Dysplasia: Alteration in the size, shape and organization of cells or tissues.

ECG: Electrocardiogram.

-ectomy: Surgical removal. For example, splenectomy is surgical removal of the spleen.

Edema: Abnormal accumulation of fluid. For example, pulmonary edema refers to a build-up of fluid in the lungs.

EFS: Event-free survival.

EKG: Electrocardiogram.

Electrocardiogram: Test to determine the pattern of a patient's heartbeat.

Electrolyte: Minerals found in the blood such as potassium that must be maintained within a certain range to prevent organ malfunction.

Emesis: Vomiting.

-emia: Of the blood. Usually refers to a blood disorder, e.g., leukemia or anemia.

Encephalopathy: Abnormal functioning of the brain.

Enzyme: A protein that is capable of triggering a chemical reaction.

Esophagitis: Inflammation of the throat.

Febrile: Pertaining to fever.

Foley catheter: Flexible plastic tube inserted into the bladder to provide continuous urinary drainage.

Gastritis: Inflammation of the stomach.

Gastrointestinal: Refers to the stomach and intestines.

Gene: A unit of genetic material that carries the directions a cell uses to perform a specific function, such as making a given protein.

Glucose: A sugar found in blood.

Hb: Hemoglobin.

HBV: Hepatitis B virus.

HCT: Hematopoietic cell transplantation.

HCV: Hepatitis C virus.

HD: Hodgkin lymphoma.

Hematology: The study of blood and its disorders.

Hematopoiesis: The formation and development of blood cells, usually takes place in the bone marrow.

Hematopoietic cells: Cells from which all blood cells derive.

Hemoglobin: The part of red blood cells that carries oxygen to tissues.

Hemorrhage: Bleeding.

Hemorrhagic cystitis: Bladder ulcers.

Hepat (o): Pertaining to the liver.

HHV6: Human herpes virus 6.

HL: Hodgkin lymphoma.

Hyper-: Excessive, increased.

Hyperal: Hyperalimentation.

Hyperalimentation: supplying nutrients intravenously.

Hyperpigmentation: Darkening of the skin.

Hypertension: High blood pressure.

Hypo-: A deficiency, less than usual.

Hypotension: Low blood pressure.

i.m.: intramuscular.

Immune complex: A cluster of interlocking antigens and antibodies.

Immune response: The reactions of the immune system to foreign substances.

Immunocompetent: Capable of developing an immune response.

Immunocompromised: A condition in which the immune system is not functioning normally.

Immunoglobulin: An antibody.

Immunosuppression: A condition in which the patient's immune system is functioning at a lower than normal level.

Immunotoxin: A naturally occurring toxin.

Inflammatory response: Redness, warmth, swelling, pain, and loss of function produced in response to infection, as the result of increased blood flow and an influx of immune cells and secretions.

Interleukins: A major group of lymphokines and monokines.

Intramuscular: Within a muscle.

Intravenous: In a vein.

IP: Interstitial pneumonia.

-itis: Inflammation.

IV: Intravenous.

Karnofsky performance score: A measure of the patient's overall physical health, judged by his level of activity.

KPS: Karnofsky performance score.

Lactose intolerance: An inability to easily digest lactose.

Lactose: A sugar found in milk.

Laminar air flow unit: An air filtering system used at some transplant facilities to remove particulate matter and fungi from the air.

Lipids: Fats.

Low-microbial diet: Special diet designed to reduce a patient's exposure to bacteria.

Lymph nodes: Small bean-shaped organs of the immune system, distributed widely throughout the body.

Lymph: A transparent, slightly yellow fluid that carries lymphocytes, bathes the body tissues, and drains into the lymphatic vessels.

Lymphatic vessels: A body-wide network of channels, similar to the blood vessels, which transport lymph to the immune organs and into the bloodstream.

Lymphoid organs: The organs of the immune system, where lymphocytes develop and congregate. They include the bone marrow, thymus, lymph nodes, spleen, and various other clusters of lymphoid tissue. The blood vessels and lymphatic vessels can also be considered lymphoid organs.

Lymphokines: Powerful chemical substances secreted by lymphocytes. These soluble molecules help direct and regulate the immune responses.

Mab: Monoclonal antibody.

Malabsorption: Failure of intestines to properly absorb oral medications or nutrients from food.

Mentation: Thinking.

Metabolite: A by-product of the breakdown of either food or medication by the body.

Metastatic: Spread of a disease from the organ or tissue of origin to another part of the body.

Microbes: Minute living organisms, including bacteria, viruses, fungi and protozoa.

Microorganisms: Microscopic plants or animals.

Minerals: Nutrients required by the body in small amounts to maintain proper fluid balance and body function.

MM: Multiple myeloma.

Molecule: The smallest amount of a specific chemical substance that can exist alone.

Monoclonal antibodies: Antibodies that are all identical, derived from a single source.

Monokines: Powerful chemical substances secreted by some white blood cells. These soluble molecules help direct and regulate the immune responses.

Morbidity: Sickness, side effects and symptoms of a treatment or disease.

MRD: Minimal residual disease.

MRI: Magnetic resonance imaging. A method of taking pictures of body tissue using magnetic fields and radio waves.

MTD: Maximum tolerated dose.

Myeloablative: Suppresses the immune system

Natural Killer cells: Type of white blood cell that can recognize and destroy some tumor cells

Nephro-: Pertaining to the kidneys.

Neuro-: Pertaining to the nervous system.

NHL: Non-Hodgkin lymphoma.

NPO: Do not take anything by mouth.

Nutrient: The part of food you eat that's used by the body to grow, function and stay alive. Nutrients include protein, carbohydrate, minerals, fat and vitamins.

Oncology: The study of cancer.

Opportunistic infection: An infection in a person whose immune system is suppressed, caused by an organism that does not usually trouble people with healthy immune systems.

Organism: An individual living thing.

Oto-: Pertaining to the ear.

Packed red blood cells: Whole blood minus the plasma.

Palliative: Provides relief rather than a cure.

Pancytopenia: A deficiency of all types of blood cells.

Parasite: A plant or animal that lives, grows and feeds on or within another living organism.

Passive immunity: Immunity resulting from the transfer of antibodies or antiserum produced by another individual.

-pathy: Disease.

PBPC: Peripheral blood progenitor cells.

PBSC: Peripheral blood stem cells.

-penia: Deficiency. For example, neutropenia means a deficiency of a type of white blood cell called a neutrophil.

Petechiae: Small red spots on the skin that usually indicate a low platelet count.

Phlebitis: Inflammation of a vein.

-plasia: Development, formation.

PLT: Platelet.

PR: Partial remission.

Prognosis: The predicted or likely outcome.

Prophylactic: Preventive measure or medication.

Protein: One of the three nutrients that supply calories to the body. Protein helps build muscle, bone, skin and blood.

Protocol: The plan for treating the patient.

Pulmonary: Pertaining to the lungs.

QOL: Quality of life.

Reflux: A backflow of acid from the stomach into the esophagus.

Relapse: Recurrence of the disease following treatment.

Relapse-free survival: Survival after treatment without relapse.

Remission, complete: Condition in which no cancerous cells can be detected by a microscope, and the patient appears to be disease-free.

Remission, cytogenetic: In persons who had a chromosomal abnormality, a remission with normal chromosomes.

Remission, partial: Generally means that by all methods used to measure the existence of a tumor, there has been at least a 50 percent regression of the disease following treatment.

Renal: Pertaining to the kidney.

RFS: Relapse-free survival.

RSV: Respiratory syncytial virus.

S.C.: Subcutaneous.

SCLC: Small cell lung cancer.

Sepsis: The presence of organisms in the blood.

Serum: The clear liquid that separates from the blood when it is allowed to clot. This fluid retains any antibodies that were present in the whole blood.

Solid tumor: A cancer that originates in organ or tissue other than bone marrow or the lymph system.

Spleen: A lymphoid organ in the abdominal cavity that is an important center for immune system activities.

Stomatitis: Inflammation of the mouth, tongue or gums.

Subcutaneous: Under the skin.

Superinfection: An infection that occurs in a patient who already has a different type of infection.

Tandem transplant: Two planned transplants, one after another.

TBI: Total body irradiation.

Thymus: A primary lymphoid organ, high in the chest, where lymphocytes proliferate and mature.

TLC: Total lung capacity.

Toxins: Agents produced by plants and bacteria that are very damaging to human cells.

Trauma: Injury.

Tumor burden: The size of the tumor or number of abnormal cells in the organ or tissue.

Tumor: Uncontrolled growth of abnormal cells in an organ or tissue.

Ultrasound: A technique for taking a picture of internal organs or other structures using sound waves.

URI: Upper respiratory infection.

Vaccine: A substance that contains components of an infectious organism. Injecting the vaccine into a person will stimulate an immune response (but not a full case of disease), and protect the person against subsequent infection by that organism.

Whole blood: Blood that has not been separated into its various components.

Xerostomia: Dryness of the mouth caused by malfunctioning salivary glands.

INDEX

Aspergillus, 71
Ativan®, 94
Atovaquone, 71
Avascular necrosis, 132

B-cell, 150
Bacteria, 11, 69-71 75, 150
Bactrim®, 72
Basophils, 150-151, 155
Be the Match®, 3, 18
BiCNU®, 66
Bilirubin, 64
Bisphosphonate, 132
Bladder, irritation 64, 70
Blast cells, 151
Bleomycin, 133
Blood and Marrow Transplant Information Network
    Caring Connections Peer Support, ix
    Survivorship Symposium, 181
    Web Site, viii
Blood cells,
    Types of, 5-6, 149-151
    Tests to measure, 153-155
Blood transfusion, 11
BMT (see Bone marrow, transplant)
BMT InfoNet (see Blood and Marrow Transplant Information Network)
Bone health, 122, 127, 132
Bone marrow,
    Aspirate (biopsy), 50, 93-94
    Definition, 5
    Harvest, 9-10
    Transplant, 3, 6
Bortezomib, 134
Breathing problems, 65
Brentuximab, 133
Busulfan, 62, 64

C. Diff, 87

Cancer, after transplant, 135

Candida, infection, 71

Caregiver, 12, 22-23, 41, 55, 103-104, 106-109, 112-114, 128

Caring Connections Program, ix

Carmustine, 64, 66, 133

Cataracts, 122, 132

Catheter, 159

  Apheresis, 8, 10, 60, 62

  Central venous, 10, 104, 159

  Foley, 161

Caverject®, 140

CBC (see complete blood count)

CBT (see Cognitive behavioral therapy)

CBT-I (see Cognitive behavioral therapy, for insomnia)

Center for International Blood & Marrow Transplant Research, 25, 122

Central venous catheter, 8, 10, 104, 159

Cerubidine®, 137

Chemotherapy,

  High-dose, 1, 2, 4, 6, 10, 61-62

  Side effects, 38, 49, 62-67, 82, 83, 85-88, 93, 137, 140-142

Children, having after transplant,

  Adoption, 146-147

  Medically assisted reproduction 143-147

Children's Oncology Group, 122

Cialis®, 140

CIBMTR (see Center for International Blood & Marrow Transplant Research)

Cisplatin, 134

Clostridium difficile colitis, 87

CMV (see Cytomegalovirus)

Cognitive behavioral therapy, 130-132

  For insomnia, 131

Cognitive problems after transplant, 128

  Attention/concentration, lack of, 127-128, 130, 136

  Confusion, 12, 65, 66

Fatigue, 127-130
Fertility after transplant, 67, 134, 136-137, 143-146
Filgrastim, 8 (see also Growth factors)
Financial assistance, 23-25
  Accelerated life insurance benefits, 30-31
  Fundraising, 31-32
  Viatical settlements, 30-31
Fluconazole, 71
Fluid retention, 64
Fluoride rinses, 134
Foley catheter, 161
Foundation for Accreditation of Cellular Therapy, 18

G-CSF (see Growth factors)
Ganciclovir, 72
Groshong® catheter (see Central venous catheter)
Growth factors, 11, 94
Growth problems in children, 128, 135-136, 166

Hair loss, 38, 64
Health Resources & Services Administration, 18
Heart problems, 66, 127, 130, 133, 137
Hematopoietic, 1, 161
Hemoglobin, 153-154, 161
Hemorrhagic cystitis, 161
Hepatitis, 161
Herbs, safety of, 80, 89-90, 133
Herpes simplex virus (HSV), 72-73
Herpes zoster (see Varicella zoster virus)
Hickman® catheter (see Central venous catheter)
Hormone deficiency, 129
  Bones and, 132
  Fatigue and, 129
  Growth and, 136
  Sexual health and, 132, 141
  Thyroid, 136

HPV (see Human papilloma virus)
HSV (see Herpes simplex virus)
Human papilloma virus, 74
Hydromorphone, 92
Hyperalimentation, 81, 161
Hyperpigmentation, 64, 161
Hypnosis, 93, 95, 98, 100

ICSI (see Intracytoplasmic sperm injection)
Ifosfamide, 64
IL-6, 129
Imodium®, 88
In-vitro fertilization (IVF), 144-145
Infection,
   Aspergillus, 71
   Bacterial, 70-71
   Candida, 71
   Fungal, 71-72
   Hepatitis, 161
   Herpes simplex virus (HSV), 72-73
   Herpes zoster, (see Varicella zoster virus)
   Human papilloma virus (HPV), 74
   Pneumocystis carinii, 72
   Pneumocystis jirovecii, 72
   Preventing, 11, 75
   Varicella Zoster Virus (VZV), 73-74
Infertility, 66-67, 134, 143-147
   Discussing with teens, 49
Insomnia (see Sleep)
Insurance, 17, 23-24, 27-31, 145
Interferon, 129
Intracytoplasmic sperm injection (ICSI), 144
Isavuconazonium sulfate, 71
IVF (see In-vitro fertilization)

Jaundice, 64
Joint deterioration, 132

Kepivance®, 63
Kidneys,
   Damage, herbs and supplements 89
   Disease, 133
   Fluid retention, 65
   Infection, 74
KY Liquibeads™ 141

Lactaid®, 88
Lactose intolerance, 87
Lenalidomide, 134
Leukemia & Lymphoma Society, The , 32
Leukocytes, 5, 149
Levitra®, 140
Lidocaine®, 63, 93
Life insurance, accelerated benefits, 29-31
Liver,
   Abnormal blood test, 64
   Cytomegalovirus, 74
   Effect of herbs, botancials and supplements on, 89
   Fluid retention, 64
   Infection, 74-75
   Jaundice, 64
   Sinusoidal Obstruction Syndrome (SOS), 65
   Toxoplasmosis, 75
Long-term health, 24-25, 120-122
Lungs,
   Breathing difficulty, 65
   Bronchitis, 70
   Infection, 71-75, 66
   Pulmonary function tests, 7, 122
   Scarring in, 133

Autologous Stem Cell Transplants: A Handbook for Patients

Sinusoidal Obstruction Syndrome, 65
Lymphocyte, 150, 157

Maintenance therapy, 135
Marital Relationships, 45, 54-55, 124-125
Massage, 93, 98, 101
MCH (see Mean corpuscular hemoglobin)
MCHC (see Mean corpuscular hemoglobin concentration)
MCV (see Mean corpuscular volume)
Mean corpuscular hemoglobin, 154
Mean corpuscular hemoglobin concentration, 154
Mean corpuscular volume, 154
Melphalan, 133
Memory problems, 123, 127-130
Menopause, premature, 136, 141
Mepron®. 72
Mesna, 64
Mesnex® (see Mesna)
Metoclopramide, 87
Mitoxantrone, 137
Monocytes, 150-151
Morphine, 63, 73, 91-93
Mouth, (see also Eating)
    Dry, 81, 83, 122, 137
    Eating difficulties, 82-90
    Sores, 12, 38, 63-64, 82-83, 93, 96
Mozobil®, 8
Mucositis (see Mouth, sores)
Muscle,
    Contractions, 63
    Cramps, 66
    Infection, 75
    Pain, 94
    Spasms, 66
    Tightness, 63

Narcotics, 63, 97

Nausea,
  Conditioning regimen side effect, 62-63
  During stem cell collection, 8
  While eating, 85-86
Nebupent®, 72
Nerve damage (see Neuropathy)
Neupogen®, 8
Neuropathy, peripheral, 94-95, 127, 134
Neutrophil, 155, 157, 164
Noxafil®, 71
Nutrition, 38, 79-90, 129

Opioid, 89, 92-96
Osteoporosis, 122, 132
Ovarian failure, 136, 141

Pain,
  Children, preparing for, 49-50
  Eating, during, 82-83
  Intercourse, during, 141
  Medication, 91-102, 96-97
  Non-drug methods of relief, 97-101
  Patient controlled analgesia machine (PCA), 97
  Peripheral neuropathy, 94-95, 127, 134
  Specialist, finding a, 101-102
  Varizella Zoster Virus (shingles), 73
Palifermin, 63
Papovavirus, 74
Parenteral nutrition, 81
PBSC (see Peripheral blood stem cell)
Pediatric transplant patients, 21, 45-60
  Dental Problems, 137
  Growth after transplant, 135
  Heart problems, 137
  Helping cope emotionally, 114

Respiratory syncytial virus (RSV), 74
Revlimid®, 134
Ribavirin, 74
Ritalin®, 130
RSV (see Respiratory syncytial virus)

Saliva,
  lack of, 83-84, 134
  thick, 84
Secondary Cancers, 135
Sedatives, 39, 62
Septra®, 72
Sexual health after transplant, 134, 139-142
Shingles (see Varicella zoster virus)
Shingrix, 74
Siblings,
  Care during transplant, 54
  Emotional concerns, 45, 50, 57-59
  Preparing for transplant, 48
Silvaderm®, 93
Sinusoidal obstruction syndrome (SOS), 65
Skin,
  Dark spots, 64
  Rash, 64, 73
Sleep difficulties, 39-40, 130-132
  Cognitive behavioral therapy for, 131
Smoking, 133
Society for Behavioral Sleep Medicine, 131
SOS (see Sinusoidal obstruction syndrome)
Sperm banking, 66-67, 143-144
Stem cell
  Collection/harvest, 7-9
  Role of, 5
Stomatitis (see Throat sores)
Substance abuse, 55, 130
Support group, 44, 126

Umbilical cord blood transplant, 1
Urination, painful, 64

Vaccination after transplant, 77-78, 122
Vaginal dryness, 141
Valcyclovir, 73
Valtrex®, 73
Varicella zoster virus (VZV), 72-73
Velcade®, 134
Veno-occlusive disease (see Sinusoidal obstruction syndrome)
Versed®, 94
Vfend®, 71
Viagra®, 140
Viatical settlement, 30-31
Vincristine, 134
Virazole®, 74
Virus, 11, 150, 163
    Adenovirus, 74
    Cytomegalovirus (CMV), 74
    Herpes simplex virus, 72-73
    Herpes zoster virus (see Varicella zoster virus)
    Human papilloma virus, 74
    Epstein-Barr virus, 74
    Papovavirus, 74
    Respiratory syncytial virus, 74, 165
    Varicella zoster virus, 73-74
VOD (see Sinusoidal obstruction syndrome)
Vomiting, 12, 62-63, 81, 85
Voriconazole®, 71
VZV (see Varicella zoster virus)

WBC (see White blood cell, count)
WBC differential, (see White blood cell, differential)
Weight, 64, 80, 86
White blood cells, 149-151, 154, 155

Celebrating a Second Chance at Life Survivorship Symposium!

BMT InfoNet's **Celebrating a Second Chance at Life Survivorship Symposium** provides a unique opportunity for survivors and their loved ones to learn how to manage the many medical, psychosocial and financial issues that can arise after transplant.

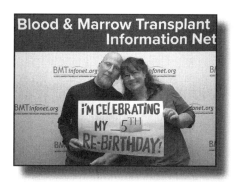

> *"This is the BEST single-point resource for survivors to get accurate and current information about their long-term side effects. I felt like the heavens opened up when I attended the Survivorship Symposium in Chicago."*
>
> *Claudia, transplant survivor*

We would love to meet you at the next Celebrating a Second Chance at Life Survivorship Symposium.

Email help@bmtinfonet.org or phone 888-597-7674 if you would like to be notified when the next symposium will occur.

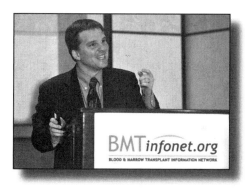

Notes

Autologous Stem Cell Transplants: A Handbook for Patients

Notes

Notes

Notes

Notes

Autologous Stem Cell Transplants: A Handbook for Patients